Recent Advances in Dentistry
(Volume 1)
Orthodontic Biomechanics:
Treatment of Complex Cases
Using Clear Aligner

Authored By

Tarek El-Bialy
Faculty of Medicine and Dentistry
University of Alberta
Edmonton, Alberta T6G 2E
Canada

Donna Galante
6526 Lonetree Blvd. Suite 100
Rocklin, CA 95765
USA

&

Sam Daher
Daher Orthostyle
1555 Marine Dr #204
West Vancouver, BC V7V 1H9
Canada

Recent Advances in Dentistry

Volume # 1

Orthodontic Biomechanics: Treatment of Complex Cases Using Clear Aligner

Authors: Tarek El-Bialy, Donana Galante & Sam Daher

ISSN (Online): 2468-5046

ISSN (Print): 2468-5038

ISBN (eBook): 978-1-68108-311-7

ISBN (Print): 978-1-68108-312-4

advertisements or ideas contained in the Work.

Limitation of Liability:

In no event will Bentham Science Publishers, its staff, editors and/or authors, be liable for any damages, including, without limitation, special, incidental and/or consequential damages and/or damages for lost data and/or profits arising out of (whether directly or indirectly) the use or inability to use the Work. The entire liability of Bentham Science Publishers shall be limited to the amount actually paid by you for the Work.

General:

1. Any dispute or claim arising out of or in connection with this License Agreement or the Work (including non-contractual disputes or claims) will be governed by and construed in accordance with the laws of the U.A.E. as applied in the Emirate of Dubai. Each party agrees that the courts of the Emirate of Dubai shall have exclusive jurisdiction to settle any dispute or claim arising out of or in connection with this License Agreement or the Work (including non-contractual disputes or claims).
2. Your rights under this License Agreement will automatically terminate without notice and without the need for a court order if at any point you breach any terms of this License Agreement. In no event will any delay or failure by Bentham Science Publishers in enforcing your compliance with this License Agreement constitute a waiver of any of its rights.
3. You acknowledge that you have read this License Agreement, and agree to be bound by its terms and conditions. To the extent that any other terms and conditions presented on any website of Bentham Science Publishers conflict with, or are inconsistent with, the terms and conditions set out in this License Agreement, you acknowledge that the terms and conditions set out in this License Agreement shall prevail.

Bentham Science Publishers Ltd.
Executive Suite Y - 2
PO Box 7917, Saif Zone
Sharjah, U.A.E.
Email: subscriptions@benthamscience.org

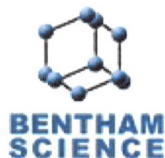

BENTHAM SCIENCE

CONTENTS

FOREWORD

Clear aligner therapy is one of the exciting new techniques being used in orthodontics since it was introduced in the late 1990s by Align Technology in the United States. Recently, other companies have come out with products that use a similar principle, but incorporate a different technology and use different materials. Aligner treatment was initially introduced to treat limited malocclusion and/or relapsed cases.

In recent years, there have been a number of articles about the use of clear aligners in a broader spectrum of orthodontic cases than just simple crowding or relapse cases. These publications and presentations focus more on treatment outcomes than on the related diagnosis process, treatment planning and biomechanics.

Understanding three-dimensional diagnosis and treatment planning as well as biomechanics of tooth movement are very important to clinicians who may use clear aligners to treat difficult orthodontic cases. This book outlines basic principles for using clear aligners to address various difficult orthodontic cases.

Dr. Jae Hyun Park
Arizona School of Dentistry & Oral Health
5835 East Still Circle
Mesa, AZ 85206
USA
Tel: 480-248-8165
Fax: 480-248-8117
Email: JPark@atsu.edu

PREFACE

The introduction of clear aligners in orthodontics as a treatment modality for complex and difficult cases has gained a worldwide acceptance/attention nowadays due to the increased advantages over regular fixed orthodontic systems. These advantages include, but not limited to the following; 1) Clear aligners are more esthetically acceptable than fixed orthodontic braces including clear (Ceramic or plastic systems) due to the fact that even with regular clear braces, metal wires are still being used which usually are seen from a distance and Teflon coated wires usually undergo peeling off the Teflon coat, which leads to the wire metal be seen; 2) clear aligners require less maintenance compared to regular fixed appliances, in other words, less emergency visits like broken brackets, poking wires and other associated complications with regular fixed orthodontic braces; 3) no food restriction like with clear aligners usually as with regular fixed orthodontic braces since the patients remove the aligners during meals and eat normally, brush and floss normally then wear the aligners back; 4) no human error in bracket positioning like those in regular fixed orthodontic braces. Even with sophisticated computerized indirect bonding techniques that utilize sophisticated computer softwares for bracket positioning with fixed orthodontic braces, most of the time the clinician has to do wire bending and normally finishing fixed orthodontic cases takes at least six to eight months on average, mainly to fix minor human errors in bracket positioning; 5) clear aligners can be more hygienic if the patient brushes his/her teeth normally as there is no much time needed to brush and floss around brackets and wires with regular orthodontic braces, and 6) nowadays difficult and complex tooth movements can be readily obtained by clear aligners when clinicians can utilize basic understanding of orthodontic mechanics during deigning and treatment planning cases using clear aligners. Finally, even in cases with bad oral hygiene when patients may undergo severe enamel decalcification with clear aligners, the aligners can be used as fluoride applicators to help with enamel re-mineralization. This does not mean that orthodontic treatment with clear aligners does not have challenges. Main challenges in orthodontic treatment with clear aligners include but not limited to the following: 1) Treatment efficacy, which could be mainly due to patients compliance, and this is not different in adults or teenagers; 2) challenges related to aligners' plastic materials which are continuously improving, however there is a lot to be done in research and development (R&D) for optimum results; 3) essential diagnosis and treatment planning of the cases which should not violate basic foundation of orthodontic skeletal/dental and esthetic evaluation and needs for each patient; 4) oral hygiene can be a problem if the patient does not maintain oral hygiene, clear aligners could act as a plaque incubator. This book is intended to present the authors' own experience with difficult cases including skeletal class I, Class II and Class III as well as facial asymmetry. However, before jumping into deep water, it may be wise to know how to swim in shallow water. This is what this book is intended to provide the reader with step by step diagnosis and treatment planning in general then introduction to biomechanics in orthodontics in general, and finally cases will be presented and discussed in terms of diagnosis, treatment planning and case management. It is also to be noted that this first edition of the book is intended to present initial cases and it is expected in the next editions that more challenging cases will be presented and their treatment planning and results will be discussed. With this, I would like to thank the contributors, all my supporting staff and family for providing support in documenting these cases and also I would like to dedicate this work to my family who sacrificed long hours and days of family time so I can finish this book.

ACKNOWLEDGEMENTS

Declared none.

CONFLICT OF INTEREST

The authors of this book testify that they do not have any conflict of interest with any clear aligner company. Also, the authors do not promote any specific clear aligner company or favor one company over the others. Again, the authors present their own cases without claiming any financial rewards from any company.

Dr. Tarek El-Bialy
Faculty of Medicine and Dentistry
7-020D Katz Group Centre for Pharmacy and Health Research
University of Alberta, Edmonton, Alberta T6G 2E
Canada
Tel: 780-492-2751, Fax: 780-492-7536
Email: telbialy@ualberta.ca

Dr. Donna Galante
6526 Lonetree Blvd. Suite 100, Rocklin, CA 95765
USA
Tel: 916-287-0078
Email: drgalante@gmail.com
&
Dr. Sam Daher
Daher Orthostyle, 1555 Marine Dr #204, West Vancouver, BC V7V 1H9
Canada
Tel: +1 604-913-1555
Email: drdaher@orthostyle.com

CHAPTER 1

Introduction/History of Clear Aligners

Abstract: Orthodontic treatment without braces has been introduced more than half a century before clear aligners have been introduced in orthodontics. Clear aligners have been utilized to treat minor crowding for more than a decade. However, in the last few years, there has been increased interest and many publications came out in different prestigious peer reviewed journals about the possibility of using clear aligners to treat difficult orthodontic cases. Different companies that manufacture clear aligners for orthodontic tooth movement spent a huge time span and resources to optimize treatment results and to provide more controlled tooth movement. The research and development included, but not limited to design attachments that can provide optimum tooth control, develop new plastic material that can have shape memory in order to maximize its efficiency in tooth movement and developing protocols for different malocclusions. There is a huge global interest in using clear aligners in orthodontics, however it might take decades for traditional orthodontists to adopt clear aligners in orthodontic practice. This chapter will briefly review the available literature about the background of clear aligners and its future application in orthodontics.

Keywords: Aligners, Clear, History, Invisible, Minor, Movement, Orthodontics, Relapse, Tooth.

Moving teeth without braces has been introduced long time ago by Kesling in 1945 [1] and the concept of clear retainer was reported by many authors afterwards [2 - 6]. Great interest in using clear aligners began in late 1990s when some orthodontic patients have had some relapse and two options were presented to the patients, retreatment or using a new version of clear plastic that is used to fabricate retainer, known as Essex retainer. The older version of active Essex retainer is known as spring aligner, or spring retainer, also known as Barrer retainer because it was first introduced by H.G Barrer in 1975. As it was first described by Barrer, an impression is taken, poured in stone then teeth are

Tarek El-Bialy, Donna Galante & Sam Daher

crowded or relapsed then the teeth are cut, set then the problem is fixed the patient has (mainly re-crowding) (Fig. **1**) [7].

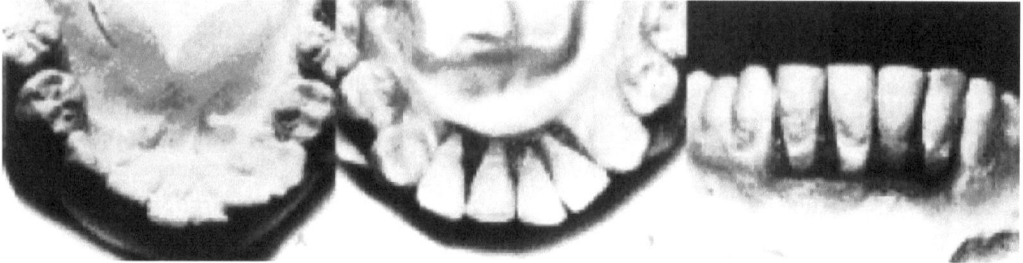

Fig. (1). Set up of the model stone to correct relapsed or crowded teeth for fabrication of spring aligners [7].

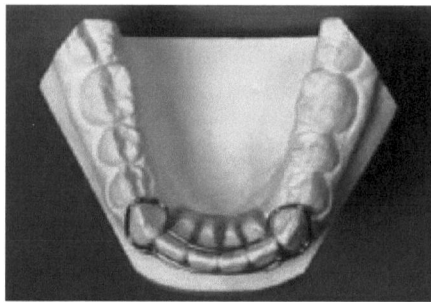

Fig. (2). Spring retainer/aligner fabricated on set stone teeth model.

Spring aligner (Fig. **2**) can be fabricated for maxillary or mandibular teeth and it was first introduced by H. G. Barrer in 1975. The mandibular appliance is mainly used today. It consists of a single piece of stainless steel wire 0.022 inch (0.56 mm) to 0.029 inch (0.72 mm) in diameter, bent around the six anterior teeth.

The spring aligner used is difficult to fabricate and hard to predict its results' outcome. When the crowding is beyond a millimeter in each contact, more than one aligner (spring aligner or Essix aligner) needs to be fabricated; this is how clear aligners started.

Not too far away, in 1993, 1994 initial reports about using Essix technology/ plastic to move teeth. [5, 8 - 10]. Sheridan philosophy is to simplify orthodontic treatment using Essix plastics and interproximal reduction, a technique that can resolve crowding as severe as to 10 mm of dental arch length deficiency and more importantly to control anchorage with other appliances [5, 8].

Invisalign or Align technology in 1999 took this idea further to utilize CAD/CAM (Computer aided design-computer aided manufacturing) technology, that can integrate digital treatment planning using clincheck software that allows the clinician to request specific tooth movement or finish and communicate this treatment planning with the technician at Invisalign. With these advances in CAD CAM technology, other companies started to appear in the market with similar technologies although the plastic used in each company could be different, and the diagnosis/treatment planning software(s) could be different between companies, the idea of utilizing clear aligners in treatment cases more than simple crowded or spaces cases can be achieved.

The first case report using Invisalign technology was presented by Boyd in 2000 for the treatment of mild crowding and space closure [11]. In a randomized clinical trial, soft and hard plastic materials were tested and changing aligners each week or two week period was also studied [12]. They concluded that all patients who completed their first set of aligners had either an additional series of case refinement aligners or fixed appliances to finish their treatment. Two-week change of aligner protocol showed a higher degree of success than 1-week change protocol. They further concluded that patients that were on the 2 week change of aligner protocol, non-extraction cases and a low PAR score were more predicted to complete their first set of aligners. Moreover, cases that had extraction treatment plans and high PAR scores showed less chances that the first set of aligners would be completed [12]. In their second study, the same group reported that the 2-week change of aligner protocol showed a larger likelihood of reduction in weighted PAR and AII scores, and higher likelihood of extraction space closure. Also, they reported that anterior alignment was the most improved part of the malocclusion, and buccal occlusion was the least improved part. They also compared treatment outcomes in lower incisor and premolar extraction. They reported that incisor extraction sites had a significantly greater likelihood of closure than any premolar extraction sites [13].

Treatment efficacy of Invisalign has been studied at different times, (2005) [14, 15] and 2009 [16], 2014 [17]. Most of the earlier reports (2005, 2009) agreed that the effectiveness of the Invisalign aligners ranged between 29.6% to 47.1% of the planned tooth movement [16]. However, the recent study by Simone *et al.* 2014 concluded that bodily tooth movements such as molar distalization, incisor torque, as well as premolar derotation can be achieved using the Invisalign® system. In addition, they concluded that the efficacy of premolar derotation depends mainly on the rate (velocity) and the total planned tooth movement. Moreover, they reported that upper incisor torque and premolar rotation are difficult types of tooth movements using removable aligners [17]. Regardless of the tremendous amount of resources invested by Align technology in research and development, it can be inferred that there is so much to learn regarding the biomechanics and efficacy of the Invisalign or similar clear aligner systems. A better understanding of the ability of clear aligner to move teeth might help the clinician to select suitable patients for treatment, monitor the proper sequencing of movement, and reduce the need for additional aligners [17].

With this brief review, it seems that understanding the biomechanics could be the key to optimize treatment results with clear aligners. Hence, the essence of this book is to review biomechanics in orthodontics and how understanding biomechanics can provide best possible orthodontic treatment results with clear aligners.

REFERENCES

[1]   Kesling HD. The philosophy of the tooth positioning appliance. Am J Orthod 1945; 31: 297-304.

[2]   Nahoum HI. The vacuum formed dental contour appliance. N Y State Dent J 1964; 9: 385-90.

[3]   Ponitz RJ. Invisible retainers. Am J Orthod 1971; 59(3): 266-72.
      [http://dx.doi.org/10.1016/0002-9416(71)90099-6] [PMID: 5276727]

[4]   McNamara JA Jr, Kramer KL, Juenker JP. Invisible retainers. J Clin Orthod 1985; 19(8): 570-8.
      [PMID: 3862671]

[5]   Sheridan JJ, LeDoux W, McMinn R. Essix retainers: fabrication and supervision for permanent retention. J Clin Orthod 1993; 27(1): 37-45.
      [PMID: 8478438]

[6]   Rinchuse DJ, Rinchuse DJ. Active tooth movement with Essix-based appliances. J Clin Orthod 1997; 31(2): 109-12.
      [PMID: 9511532]

[7]   Barrer HG. Protecting the integrity of mandibular incisor position through keystoning procedure and spring retainer appliance. J Clin Orthod 1975; 9(8): 486-94.
      [PMID: 1072074]

[8]   Sheridan JJ, Ledoux W, McMinn R. Essix technology for the fabrication of temporary anterior

bridges. J Clin Orthod 1994; 28(8): 482-6.
[PMID: 8617832]

[9]   Ballard R, Sheridan JJ. Air-rotor stripping with the Essix anterior anchor. J Clin Orthod 1996; 30(7): 371-3.
[PMID: 10356483]

[10]   Rinchuse DJ, Rinchuse DJ. Active tooth movement with Essix-based appliances. J Clin Orthod 1997; 31(2): 109-12.
[PMID: 9511532]

[11]   Boyd R, Miller RJ, Vlaskalic V. The Invisalign system in adult orthodontics: mild crowding and space closure cases. J Clin Orthod 2000; 34: 13-5.

[12]   Bollen A-M, Huang G, King G, Hujoel P, Ma T. Activation time and material stiffness of sequential removable orthodontic appliances. Part 1: Ability to complete treatment. Am J Orthod Dentofacial Orthop 2003; 124(5): 496-501.
[http://dx.doi.org/10.1016/S0889-5406(03)00576-6] [PMID: 14614415]

[13]   Clements KM, Bollen A-M, Huang G, King G, Hujoel P, Ma T. Sequential removable orthodontic appliances, effects of activation time and material stiffness. Part 2: Dental improvements. Am J Orthod Dentofacial Orthop 2003; 124: 502-8.
[http://dx.doi.org/10.1016/S0889-5406(03)00577-8] [PMID: 14614416]

[14]   Djeu G, Shelton C, Maganzini A. Outcome assessment of Invisalign and traditional orthodontic treatment compared with the American Board of Orthodontics objective grading system. Am J Orthod Dentofacial Orthop 2005; 128(3): 292-8.
[http://dx.doi.org/10.1016/j.ajodo.2005.06.002] [PMID: 16168325]

[15]   Lagravère MO, Flores-Mir C. The treatment effects of Invisalign orthodontic aligners: a systematic review. J Am Dent Assoc 2005; 136(12): 1724-9.
[http://dx.doi.org/10.14219/jada.àrchive.2005.0117] [PMID: 16383056]

[16]   Kravitz ND, Kusnoto B, BeGole E, Obrez A, Agran B. How well does Invisalign work? A prospective clinical study evaluating the efficacy of tooth movement with Invisalign. Am J Orthod Dentofacial Orthop 2009; 135(1): 27-35.
[http://dx.doi.org/10.1016/j.ajodo.2007.05.018] [PMID: 19121497]

[17]   Simon M, Keilig L, Schwarze J, Jung BA, Bourauel C. Treatment outcome and efficacy of an aligner technique--regarding incisor torque, premolar derotation and molar distalization. BMC Oral Health 2014; 14(68): 68.
[http://dx.doi.org/10.1186/1472-6831-14-68] [PMID: 24923279]

CHAPTER 2

Science and Practice of Clear Aligners

Abstract: This chapter will briefly discuss the science behind using clear aligners in orthodontics. Although fabricating aligners can be made by hand in the lab or using computer aided design/computer aided manufacturing system, the science behind using specific plastic material that has specific elasticity to move the teeth in the intended direction is still unclear and many manufacturers do not declare it as a major manufacturing or business secret. In a simple assumption, the clear aligner materials must be flexible enough to accommodate the existing tooth/teeth position and be stiff enough to move the teeth in the intended direction. Although seems simple, however it took major companies decades spending many millions of dollars on research and development to reach this particular balance. In the following section, a general review of what is available in the literature about clear aligners' materials is provided.

Keywords: Aligners, Basic science, Bio, CAD/CAM, Clear, Effectiveness, Materials, Orthodontics, Piezoelectricity, System.

Initial clear aligners fabricated to resolve simple crowded teeth due to relapse were labor intensive in doing dental stone set up for each set of aligner. When the crowded teeth require few aligners to be fabricated, a full time lab technician is required to be in each orthodontic office, or an expected lab cost of approximately $100 per set of aligner. With this, it is very costly to perform such treatment and it would be better to retreat relapsed cases with fixed orthodontic treatment. With advances in CAD/CAM system as well as the use of different plastics, many aligners may be fabricated with less lab labor however; it would require large capital for investment in research and development of computer software. In addition, challenges using CAD/CAM system as well as highly sophisticated computer software based on thousands of cases treated with traditionally fabricated aligners made huge advances in taking clear aligners to the next level

Tarek El-Bialy, Donna Galante & Sam Daher

where more difficult cases may be treated solely by clear aligners without the need to use fixed orthodontic appliance at the beginning or at the end of the cases to finish and detail the occlusion. Although the author of this book is not directly or indirectly involved in any clear aligner companies, however he has been using clear aligners in the last ten years from simple to very difficult cases.

It was hypothesized that the clear plastic that has been used initially with Essex retainers may be used solely for the treatment of difficult cases without the need for fixed orthodontic appliances at any stage of the treatment. This hypothesis is based on understanding basic orthodontic diagnosis/treatment planning and mechanics in a different way to fully execute orthodontic treatment by clear aligners.

There is no much information in the literature about the chemical composition of the plastics that are being used by different companies, including Essix, Invisalign and others to improve treatment outcome in terms of flexibility and stiffness of the plastics. This could be due to the market competition and manufacturing secrets that most companies prefer not to declare in scientific literature.

In reviewing the ideal characteristics of orthodontic wires, three main properties are needed. 1) Appropriate stiffness to minimize breakage or failure during treatment by patient handling or masticatory forces; 2) Appropriate flexibility so that wire can be tied to severely crowded teeth without permanent deformation, and 3) high range of activation so that the patient can be seen over longer intervals without the need to frequent changing their wires. Similar physical properties may be needed with clear aligners. Appropriate stiffness is required to minimize breakage of the aligners due to treatment or biting on the aligners by patients, especially in weak areas where severe crowded teeth are aggregated. Also, appropriate flexibility and shape memory of clear aligners are very important so that the aligner material can be easily flexed around severely crowded teeth and can easily grasp the crowded teeth or teeth with bulbous morphology with high areas of contour. In the event that the material does not flex enough to satisfy the above mentioned criteria, it is difficult to move teeth with clear plastic aligners. Finally, it would be an ideal property that the clear aligners material possess high range of activation or shape memory such that few aligners may be used to move the teeth gradually at a lower physiological rate without applying too much force that may be deleterious to the periodontal ligament and alveolar bone.

Although different companies utilizing clear aligners and may be holding different patents on the composition and properties of the plastics that every company is using to fabricate orthodontic aligners, it seems to the author of this book that no such combination of these physical properties exists, at least at the current time, or provided by any of the current clear aligners companies.

A recent study evaluated physical properties of aged and retrieved Invisalign aligners [1]. The authors evaluated the aligners' structures after being used for two weeks by patients or aging in retrieved aligners. They reported that the retrieved aligners showed morphological changes compared to the as-received samples including abrasion at the cusp tips, adsorption of integuments, and localized calcification of the precipitated biofilm at areas of food stagnation. The authors also reported that buccal segments of retrieved aligners showed an increase in hardness, which the authors attributed this phenomenon to mastication-induced cold work, however this concept has not been explained in detail. The authors also commented that the clinical implication of this problem on treatment efficacy of Invisalign outcome is unknown as it has not been studied at this time. Since this study has been published in 2004, only recently Align technology reported to introduce a new plastic material that has improved physical and structural properties. However, again there is no much information available about the chemical composition of these new plastic materials.

An interesting, however has been overlooked, publication in 2003 when it has been shown for the first time that the plastic that has been used to fabricate Essex aligners/retainers has in fact a piezoelectric property and may be used as ultrasound transducers [2]. This property may be important in orthodontic treatment using these types of plastics and future research may be directed to improve such property of the newly developed plastic. One might ask why this piezoelectric property is important in orthodontic treatment. One of the fundamental theories of biology of orthodontic tooth movement is the piezoelectric theory [2]. According to Proffit [3], piezoelectricity is a phenomenon observed in many crystalline materials in which a deformation of the crystal structure produces a flow of electric current as electrons are displaced from one part of the crystal lattice to another. Organic crystals can also be piezoelectric, and collagen in the PDL is an excellent example. Dr. Proffit further added "Both of these characteristics are explained by the migration of electrons within the crystal lattice as it is distorted by pressure" [3]. When the crystal structure is deformed, electrons migrate from one location to another and an electric current flow is observed. As long as the force is maintained, the crystal structure is stable and no further electric events are observed. When the force is released, however, the crystal returns to its original shape, and a reverse flow of electrons is seen. With this arrangement, rhythmic activity would produce a constant interplay of current flow in one direction and then the other that would be measured as microamperes, whereas occasional application and release of force would produce only occasional signal of this type). Putting the above mentioned information together with the fact that the plastic used in clear aligners/retainers might have piezoelectric property, when the patient bite on the aligners, it is expected that these aligners might produce a flow of electric current that could help in either tooth movement and /or bone remodeling. It might be interesting to mention that it has been reported that ultrasound can minimize orthodontically induced tooth root resorption and enhances dental tissue formation [4 - 9]. Also, ultrasound enhances bone formation and maturation [10 - 12].

It might be inferred from the aforementioned literature that clear aligner plastics if possess piezoelectric properties, could enhance tooth movement and may also prevent teeth root resorption while enhancing bone remodeling. If this is true, clear aligners may push the ordinary known envelop of tooth movement limits to take it beyond traditional expectation.

Although different companies may claim inventing or improving the plastic type to have less wear, more predicted tooth movement or more flexibility, in the author's opinion piezoelectricity of the plastic used for construction of aligners is the future area of research and development.

REFERENCES

[1]   Schuster S, Eliades G, Zinelis S, Eliades T, Bradley TG. Structural conformation and leaching from *in vitro* aged and retrieved Invisalign appliances. Am J Orthod Dentofacial Orthop 2004; 126(6): 725-8. [http://dx.doi.org/10.1016/j.ajodo.2004.04.021] [PMID: 15592222]

[2]   Tawfik A, Hemeda OM, El-Bialy TH. Composite polymers transducers for ultrasonic and biological applications. Ferroelectrics Letters 2003; 30(1-2): 1-12.
[http://dx.doi.org/10.1080/713931703]

[3]   Proffit WR, Fields HW. Contemporary Orthodontics. 5th ed. Mosby 2013; p. 281.

[4]   El-Bialy T, Alhadlaq A, Lam B. Effect of therapeutic ultrasound on human periodontal ligament cells for dental and periodontal tissue engineering. Open Dent J 2012; 6: 235-9.
[http://dx.doi.org/10.2174/1874210601206010235] [PMID: 23308087]

[5]   Al-Daghreer S, Doschak M, Sloan AJ, *et al.* Long term effect of low intensity pulsed ultrasound on a human tooth slice organ culture. Arch Oral Biol 2012; 57(6): 760-8.
[http://dx.doi.org/10.1016/j.archoralbio.2011.11.010] [PMID: 22138259]

[6]   El-Bialy T, Lam B, Aldaghreer S, Sloan AJ. The effect of low intensity pulsed ultrasound in a 3D ex vivo orthodontic model. J Dent 2011; 39(10): 693-9.
[http://dx.doi.org/10.1016/j.jdent.2011.08.001] [PMID: 21856368]

[7]   Mostafa NZ, Uludag H, Dederich DN, Doschak MR, El-Bialy TH. Anabolic effects of low intensity pulsed ultrasound on gingival fibroblasts. Archives of Oral Biology 2009; 54(8): 743-48.

[8]   El-Bialy T, El-Shamy I, Graber TM. Repair of orthodontically induced root resorption by ultrasound in humans. Am J Orthod Dentofacial Orthop 2004; 126(2): 186-93.
[http://dx.doi.org/10.1016/j.ajodo.2004.02.010] [PMID: 15316473]

[9]   el-Bialy TH, el-Moneim Zaki A, Evans CA. Effect of ultrasound on rabbit mandibular incisor formation and eruption after mandibular osteodistraction. Am J Orthod Dentofacial Orthop 2003; 124(4): 427-34.
[http://dx.doi.org/10.1016/S0889-5406(03)00408-6] [PMID: 14560274]

[10]   El-Bialy TH, Royston TJ, Magin RL, Evans CA, Zaki Ael-M, Frizzell LA. The effect of pulsed ultrasound on mandibular distraction. Ann Biomed Eng 2002; 30(10): 1251-61.
[http://dx.doi.org/10.1114/1.1529196] [PMID: 12540201]

[11]   El-Bialy T, El-Shamy I, Graber TM. Growth modification of the rabbit mandible using therapeutic ultrasound: is it possible to enhance functional appliance results? Angle Orthod 2003; 73(6): 631-9.
[PMID: 14719726]

[12]   El-Bialy TH, Elgazzar RF, Megahed EE, Royston TJ. Effects of ultrasound modes on mandibular osteodistraction. J Dent Res 2008; 87(10): 953-7.
[http://dx.doi.org/10.1177/154405910808701018] [PMID: 18809750]

CHAPTER 3

Orthodontic Diagnosis and Treatment Planning

Abstract: Orthodontic treatment planning is essential before deciding what type of orthodontic treatment may be used to treat different cases. Before the development of various orthodontic appliances (standard edgewise, straight wire, self-ligating fixed bracket systems or clear aligners) one should keep in mind what are the patient's problem list, treatment objectives and treatment planning, then based on the treatment planning, mechanics can be proposed and then one can choose or not use specific appliance based on the clinician's level of comfort using such appliance. This chapter will briefly review the contemporary steps in diagnosis and treatment planning of orthodontic cases disregarding the type of tooth movement.

Keywords: CBCT, Cephalometric, Diagnosis, Model, Orthodontics, Planning, Tooth movement, Treatment, Type, X-ray.

The first reported three dimensional diagnosis and orthodontic treatment planning of complex malocclusion with the Invisalign appliance was reported by Boyd and Vlaskalic in 2001 [1]. Although this publication laid out the foundation for Invisalign or clear aligners' diagnosis and treatment planning, continuous development of diagnostic tools like con-beam-computed-tomography (CBCT) for example has enhanced and provided tremendous insights into case diagnosis and treatment planning [2]. Also, the recent introduction of intraoral cameras and scanners that can provide the clinician with immediate digital model, compared to the traditional plaster study casts, can help the clinicians to make immediate informed decision rather than taking long time to work up the cases.

Contemporary orthodontic diagnosis and treatment planning include obtaining of the following records:

Tarek El-Bialy, Donna Galante & Sam Daher

1. Patient's history (Medical and dental)
2. Patient's chief complaint
3. Clinical examination
4. Models (plaster or digital)
5. Radiographic evaluation

PATIENT'S HISTORY (MEDICAL AND DENTAL)

Obtaining patient's history (medical and dental) is of utmost importance. I would like to stress on the following questions to the new or transferred patient:

a. Do you take any medication? If so what medication(s) are you currently taking now? The importance of this question is that, it can discover any underlying systemic illnesses that might affect your decision in terms of treatment planning for the patient. For example, if the patient is under corticosteroid for allergies or asthma, the orthodontist should be aware that corticosteroid affects bone remodeling and consequently orthodontic movement which is tightly linked to duration of treatment. Most new patients will ask the following question (how much time I will be in treatment) and the orthodontist should provide a reasonable answer, without commitment to specific duration. For example, it might be advisable based on the clinician's experience to provide the new patient with a range of treatment time instead of locking himself/herself in specific time by saying (your treatment will take 18 months) it is better to say (cases like your case usually take in my hands 18 months on average depending on how compliant the patient is with my given instructions and also it depends on patients' teeth and bone response to treatment).

b. Dental history is very important to know if the patient had severe dental trauma, root canal treatment, maintaining regular checkup visits with his/her dentist or not. The importance of this information in orthodontic treatment planning includes that in patients that have had trauma to their teeth, tooth mobility and root resorption might be expected. If the patient is maintaining his/her checkup visits to the dentist, this may reflect expected good oral hygiene. Towards the end of this book, I will present a case of bad oral hygiene that led to severe decalcification under the aligners and will discuss this at the end of this book.

PATIENT'S CHEIF COMPLAINT: Although the orthodontist might see different dental or orthodontic problems in the patient's mouth upon clinical examination or after analyzing the patient's records, it is very important to investigate patients' main concerns and address them during the consultation or during the treatment. Patients with unaddressed concerns might not be happy or the clinician may lose the patients' compliance which can affect the patient's results. In order to explore this chief complaint or concern for the patient, the following question is a traditional one: Why you are here today? Or what brought you up here today?

CLINICAL EXAMINATION: This includes extra oral (profile to check if it is straight, convex or concave), this provides information about whether the patient might have skeletal class I, II or III. Also facial form (brachyfacial, mesofacial or dolichofacial type) to put into consideration the followings: If the patient is brachyfacial type, tooth movement might be difficult due to the fact that brachyfacial type patients usually have strong musculature that normally interferes with changing the occlusal pattern by orthodontic treatment. However, it may be interesting here to say that even with brachyfacial type patients, the use of clear aligners disengage the occlusion by the occlusal coverage of the teeth by plastic that can facilitate tooth movement due to minimized teeth inter-digitation.

On the other hand, dolichocephalic patients might have other problems like open bite. Also, if there is moderate to severe crowding in dolichofacial type cases, it is difficult to expand or distalize molars in these cases as these types of tooth movement can lead to exaggeration of the patient's increased vertical dimension which might result in unacceptable results. It may also be worth mentioning here that in cases of open bite, occlusal coverage of teeth by clear aligners may serve as posterior bite plate that can help with controlling the vertical dimension of the patient.

Clinical examination of the patient's facial symmetry is very important to differentiate between the patients that might require surgical intervention to improve patient's asymmetric face/chin and consequently coordinated orthodontic-orthognathic treatment planning or patient that might have lateral mandibular shift due to dental interference or bilateral constricted upper arch.

Also, extra-oral clinical examination includes type of breathing as mouth breathers are usually have constricted upper arch and wide lower arch due to the unsupported upper posterior teeth from the lingual side against the inward forces of the cheek muscles. Mouth breathing should be handled first or during orthodontic treatment to minimize the possibility of relapse after treatment due to sustained inward pressure of cheek muscles on the upper posterior teeth with no or minimum tongue support for the palatal side to the upper posterior teeth.

Intraoral examination includes centric relation-centric occlusion relationship and if there is any functional shift of the mandible upon closure (anterior, posterior or lateral shift). Identification of these shifts upon clinical examination is important in predicting difficulty or simplicity of the presented case. More details about the incorporation of these possible shifts in treatment planning and results will be presented in the section of facial asymmetry as well as in class II division 2 cases. Also, intraoral examination includes gingival health, oral hygiene, molar and canine relationships, crowding/spacing, arch width and dental midlines (upper and lower) relations as well as cross bites.

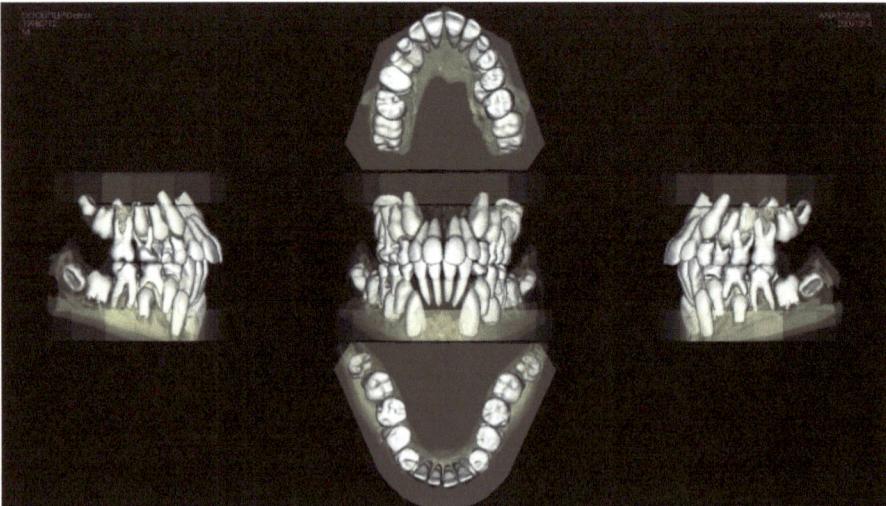

Fig. (3.1). CBCT-generated Digital model of a patient using Anatomodel software.

DENTAL STUDY MODELS (PLASTER OR DIGITAL): Dental study models are important to document the patient's initial occlusal relationships and can be used for calculating arch length deficiency as well as Bolton Discrepancy. Dental cast models can be obtained from alginate impression, constructed from initial cone-beam computed tomography (CBCT) if it is taken for the patient as an initial diagnostic radiograph. Fig. (**3.1**) below shows CBCT –generated initial digital model for a patient. Recent publications supported that digital study models generated from CBCT may be used in clinical orthodontic diagnosis and treatment planning however their use is time consuming compared to the use of dental plaster models [3].

Digital models may also be produced *via* different intraoral light/laser scanners that have been introduced to orthodontists and dental practitioners in the last two years. Some of these intraoral scanners are iTero and IOC from Cadent (Fig. **3.2**). The scanning time varies between 8 -30 minutes on average depending on the experience of the practitioner or assistants.

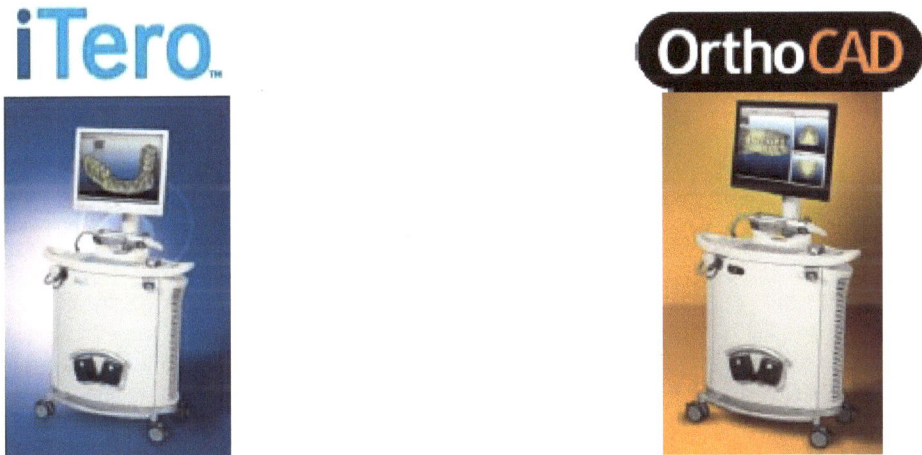

Fig. (3.2). iTero and iOC scanners.

Digital models produced from these scanners are accepted by wide manufacturers (like Invisalign) and other laboratories as well for fabrication of dental/ortho-dontic devices.

An example of the digital models generated from these scanners is in (Fig. **3.3**).

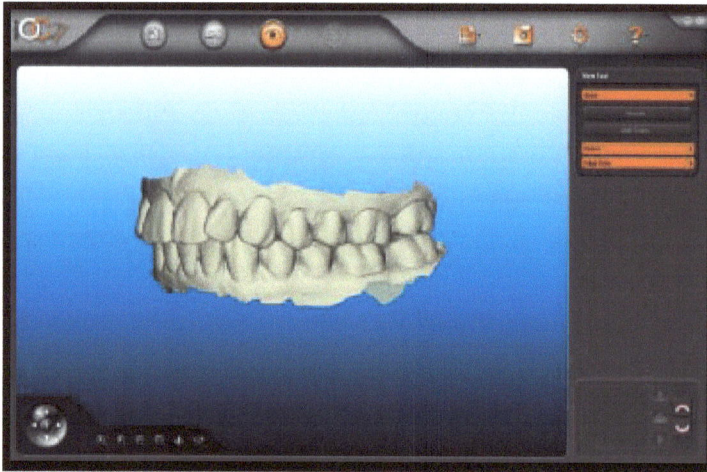

Fig. (3.3). Digital model created from iOC scanner.

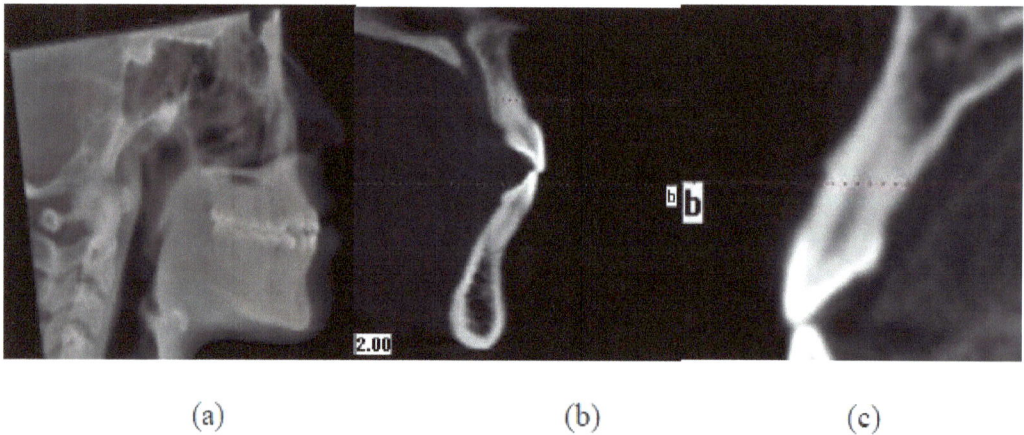

(a)   (b)   (c)

Fig. (3.4). A lateral cephalometric radiograph of a patient hardly shows the actual alveolar bone thicknesses of the anterior teeth (a). Same patient's CBCT sagittal screen shows the actual alveolar width of the anterior teeth (b). It can be seen from the cephalometric radiograph that it is impossible to estimate whether the alveolar bone widths for upper and lower incisors will be wide enough to allow for more AP movement, as yet in reality, there is not enough bone and the lower incisors do not have an adequate labial plate of bone necessary for labial tooth movement should it be required (b). The same thing applies to the upper incisors where there is inadequate labial bone to move the upper incisors labially. Labial alveolar bone height is also hard to estimate from periapical or lateral cephalometric radiographs. Only sagittal screens generated from CBCT allow for an accurate estimation of alveolar bone height (c) [2].

RADIOGRAPHIC EVALUATION: Traditional radiographic techniques that have been used in orthodontic diagnosis and treatment planning include panoramic, lateral cephalometric, full mouth periapical, postero-anterior cephalometric and sometimes tomography. However, recent publications and presentations/ discussions have shown the feasibility of performing one radiograph (CBCT) that can provide all these views with similar or less amount of radiation exposure and produces a more reliable imaging for orthodontic diagnosis and treatment planning. A recent published book has discussed these issues in details [2]. In particular alveolar bone width is very hard to estimate from regular lateral cephalometric radiographs. Alveolar bone width is extremely important especially if we are planning major anteroposterior or horizontal tooth movement. An example is shown below which shows that the symphysis width as measured from lateral cephalometric radiograph is adequate for labiolingual movement of the incisors, however the real alveolar width (labiolingually is almost half of that can be seen in lateral cephalometric radiograph (Fig. **3.4**).

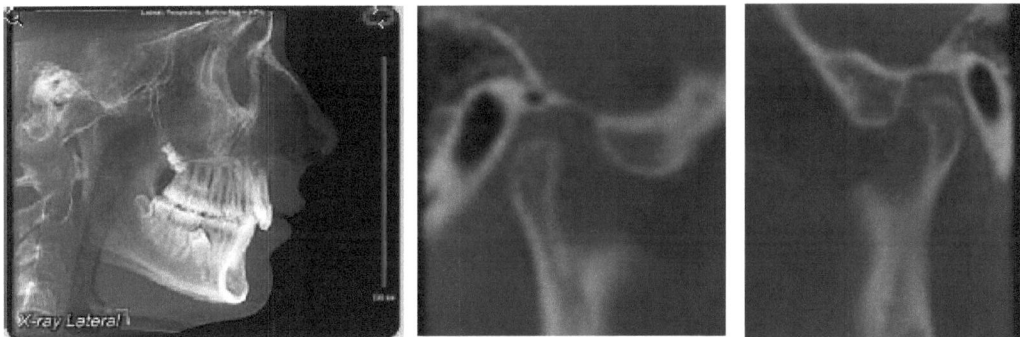

A   B

Fig. (3.5). A 15 year-old female that has skeletal Class II. A) Cephalometric x-ray shows mandibular retrognathism, however b) tomograms show distal shift of the mandible as indicated by the increased anterior disk space compared to posterior disk space. Without Tomograms, this case could have been set/planned for surgical orthodontics that may involve mandibular advancement utilizing bilateral sagittal split osteotomy. This case was finished solely by orthodontic treatment within 12 months.

Another important diagnostic image projection that can be obtained from CBCT is the temporomandibular joint (TMJ) tomograms. Whenever there is a detected clinical functional shift of the lower jaw (lateral, anterior or posterior) it should be documented radiographically in order to properly diagnose and treat such cases. Many cases will be presented in this book that initially were set for surgical orthodontics, however after careful diagnosis and documentation of lower jaw position using the TMJ tomography that has been generated from the CBCT, these cases turn out to be very simple cases and did not require any surgical intervention (Figs. **3.5**, **3.6**).

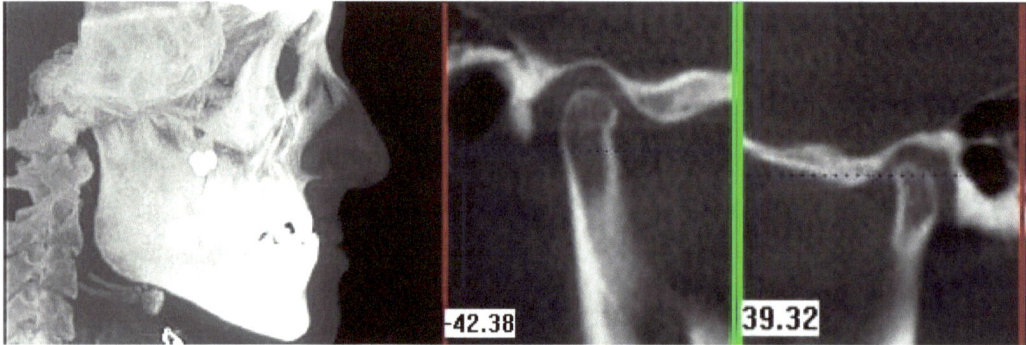

A   B

Fig. (3.6). A) Cephalometric x-ray of an adult patient presented with anterior cross bite and she was set for two jaw surgeries by another orthodontist. However, tomograms show anterior functional shift which helped planning and finishing of the case using regular orthodontic treatment non-surgically.

TMJ tomography is not only important in diagnosis and documentation of functional shift should it be speculated from clinical examination of the patients, but also it is important to document mandibular growth prediction in growing patients who may have clear aligner treatment.

It has long been acknowledged and recognized by orthodontic institutes worldwide the growth prediction studies by Bjork to help predicting mandibular growth direction [4]. One of the key factors in determining forward or backward growth direction of the mandible, according to Bjork, is the shape and direction of the mandibular condylar heads. However, none of the traditional radiographs (Lateral cephalometric and panoramic radiographs) can provide accurate estimation of the possible mandibular growth direction based on the shape of mandibular condyles. The following x-ray shows how cephalometric radiograph may not be enough to diagnose mandibular growth prediction, however tomograms confirm the forward mandibular growth tendency that can be predicted in this 15 years old male (Fig. **3.7**).

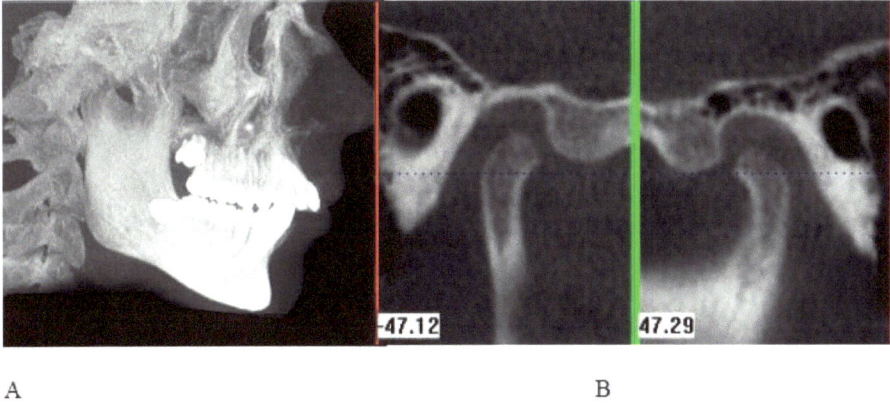

A   B

Fig. (3.7). A) Lateral cephalometric radiograph of a 15 years old male that shows severe mandibular retrognathism, however it is hard to confirm from the lateral cephalometric radiograph the shape and direction of the mandibular condyles to help predicting mandibular growth direction. B) Tomograms showing forward directed mandibular condylar heads which can help predicting forward mandibular growth even at age 15 years old boy. It can also be seen that the patient is not in full centric occlusion which also can be confirmed by Tomogram where the condyles are positioned downward and slightly forward. In addition, estimating prediction of airway size and volume cannot be predicted from regular cephalometric radiographs. CBCT or tomograms can provide an estimation of nasal and oropharyngeal airway/volume for any patients. Without documentation of this information, major etiologic factors of malocclusion like mouth breathing can be overlooked and if not managed during orthodontic treatment, relapse is most likely to occur.

Fig. (**3.8**) below shows lateral cephalometric radiograph that is very difficult to evaluate the tongue position which is very low and can be easily evaluated as well as the nasopharyngeal and oropharyngeal airway from the CBCT (Fig. **3.8**).

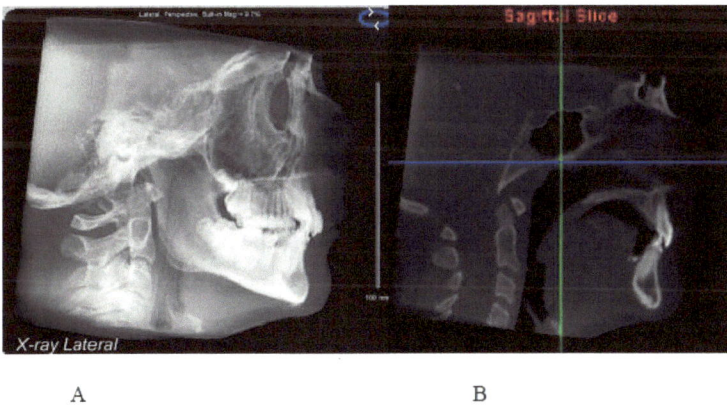

A   B

Fig. (3.8). A) Lateral cephalometric radiograph that can hardly show the tongue position or airway. B) Same patient CBCT-generated airway screen clearly shows the low/back tongue position and constricted oropharyngeal airway.

In diagnosis and treatment planning of cases with skeletal discrepancy, the concept of dental compensation should be thoroughly understood and evaluated in order to formulate better diagnosis and hence best possible treatment planning and non-compromised treatment results.

Dental compensation for skeletal discrepancy can occur in three dimensions, anteroposterior (AP), horizontal and vertical.

a. **ANTEROPOSTERIOR (AP) DENTAL COMPENSATION**: AP skeletal discrepancy can occur in the cases of class II or class III skeletal malrelationships. In the case of class II skeletal discrepancy, upper incisors are usually reteroclined while lower incisors are usually proclined. These incisors' proclination and reteroclination are dental compensation of the underlying skeletal malrelationship. The major concern with these types of dental compensation is that it is less likely that major jaw discrepancy correction may be performed without surgical intervention that usually require decompensation of the these proclined/retroclined teeth to their normal position relative to their perspective basal bones in orthodontic preparation phase before orthognathic surgery.

b. **HORIZONTAL COMPENSATION**: In severe horizontal skeletal discrepancy (for example a severely skeletal constricted maxilla relative to a normal or wide mandible), upper posterior teeth are usually tipped buccally while lower posterior teeth are tipped lingually.

In order to have a long term prognosis with healthy peridontium/alveolar bone, teeth are required to be positioned normally relative to the basal jaw bone in such a way to allow for normal distribution of occlusal forces. This requires minimizing severe tilting of teeth that normally appear as compensation for severe skeletal imbalance between upper and lower jaws.

To achieve maximum functional and esthetic results, orthodontists' goals are usually minimizing dental compensations due to skeletal malrelationship, however decompensation initially worsens the case in terms of increasing the sagittal or horizontal discrepancy (increase overjet [in skeletal class II] or increase cross bite [in skeletal class III]) until surgical correction is performed to improve skeletal malrelationship.

In summary, the author of this book Tarek El-Bialy, based on his experience with different orthodontic techniques, mechanics, and also based on his training in different countries, suggests that low radiation dose CBCT is the best way to diagnose orthodontic cases for better orthodontic treatment planning with more predictable and stable results.

REFERENCES

[1]   Boyd RL, Vlaskalic V. Three-dimensional diagnosis and orthodontic treatment of complex malocclusion with the Invisalign appliance. Semin Orthod 2001; 7: 274-93.
[http://dx.doi.org/10.1053/sodo.2001.25414]

[2]   El-Bialy T. Cone-beam computed tomography (CBCT) an essential for proper orthodontic diagnosis and treatment planning Computed Tomography: New Research. Hauppauge NY 11788-3619, USA: Nova Science Publishers, Inc. 400 Oser Ave Suite 1600 2012; pp. 241-54.

[3]   Luu NS, Nikolcheva LG, Retrouvey J-M, *et al.* Linear measurements using virtual study models. Angle Orthod 2012; 82(6): 1098-106.
[http://dx.doi.org/10.2319/110311-681.1] [PMID: 22530811]

[4]   Björk A. Prediction of mandibular growth rotation. Am J Orthod 1969; 55(6): 585-99.
[http://dx.doi.org/10.1016/0002-9416(69)90036-0] [PMID: 5253957]

CHAPTER 4

Unique Features of Clear Aligners Compared to Regular Orthodontic Appliances

Abstract: This chapter highlights the important features of clear aligners and their possible added benefit to orthodontic treatment. In particular, clear aligners disarticulate the teeth and this disarticulation makes it easy to achieve inter-arch tooth movement than with regular fixed orthodontic appliances. This chapter presents different features of clear aligners that may make tooth movement easier than fixed orthodontic appliance.

Keywords: Bite clearance, Clear aligners, Disarticulation, Early correction, Fast, Features, Orthodontics, Tooth movement, Unique.

As mentioned earlier in chapter 2 (Science and practice of clear aligners), the type of plastic that has been used to fabricate the clear aligners may have piezoelectric property which, if proven for new plastic materials, can be utilized for faster tooth movement and minimum orthodontically induced root resorption. There are other features that clear aligners may actually provide advantages over regular orthodontic braces. These features, from the author's prospective can be summarized as follows:

1. Clear aligners could be described as a short cut to predictable results compared to trial and errors when using regular braces. In other words, driving around the mountain takes longer time than taking a jet from point A to point B without hassling around the mountains. In other words, the digitally planned estimated end point (results or occlusion) can be predicted using the digital treatment plan (Clincheck for example in the case of Invisalign technology). The clinician can predict and expect how the treatment results would be wheth-

Tarek El-Bialy, Donna Galante & Sam Daher

er the patient is compliant and the patient's biological response to tooth movement is within the normal range.

2. Clear aligners allow the patients to eat sticky or hard food and better oral hygiene compared with traditional fixed orthodontic braces when patients are not allowed to eat any sticky or crunchy foods throughout the treatment otherwise brackets/tubes can be at a high risk of being broken and this would hurdle the treatment progress and might cause gum/check irritation by the broken brackets or displaced orthodontic wires due to the broken brackets. In addition, with regular fixed orthodontic braces, patients have to do meticulous tooth brushing and dental flossing around the wires and brackets/wires to minimize possible enamel decalcifications and/or periodontal disease from accumulated dental plaque around the gingival margins or in the interdental spaces if not cleaned 100%.

3. In cases of noncompliant patients, especially with retainers wear after finishing orthodontic treatment, if relapse occurs, the patient less likely requires new aligners. In the case of using fixed braces, new regular braces might be used. In fact, most likely, relapsed clear aligner cases may be able to re-use their old aligners that can reprogram their treatment towards the initially planned finished occlusions.

4. Clear aligners cover the occlusal surface of the teeth which provides many advantages that can be summarized as follows:

   a. In deep bite cases, with most likely strong musculature, tooth movement is usually restrained or difficult to achieve due to the inclined planes of posterior teeth occlusal cusps. With clear aligners, the occlusal coverage disengages the occlusion that allows for free teeth movement. It can also act as a jaw positioning splint when centric occlusion and centric relationships are not coincident.

   b. In open bite cases, the occlusal coverage of the posterior teeth by clear aligners works as posterior bite plate/block that can help in controlling the vertical dimension, especially when this is combined with anterior vertical pull chin cup.

c. In cross bite cases, the occlusal coverage of the teeth disengages the occlusion to allow easy movement of the teeth from cross bite to normal bite and this occlusal coverage works as a posterior bite plate that has long been used with removable and fixed orthodontic appliances.

d. Finally, the occlusal coverage of the posterior teeth is very important in class II cases with or without molar distalization as:

   i. In cases where molar distalization is required, occlusal coverage of posterior teeth disengages the occlusion and allows for free distal movement of upper posterior teeth.

   ii. It helps control vertical dimension and may help intrude posterior teeth, which when occurs can lead to auto-forward rotation of the mandible and consequently helps in class II correction.

5. Clear aligners are more hygienic and less gingival or periodontal problems are encountered with clear aligners when compared to either buccal or lingual fixed orthodontic appliances [1, 2].

6. The improved gingival and periodontal health can also help decrease pain with clear aligners compared to fixed orthodontic treatment [3].

7. Finally, in author's opinion, clear aligners may be used as fluoride application trays should decalcification occur during treatment due to bad oral hygiene.

It should be noted that orthodontic treatment results using clear aligners are mainly dependent on the patient's wear and compliance with the clinician's instructions.

REFERENCES

[1]   Schaefer I, Braumann B. Halitosis, oral health and quality of life during treatment with Invisalign®

and the effect of a low-dose chlorhexidine solution. J Orofac Orthop 2010; 71(6): 430-41.
[http://dx.doi.org/10.1007/s00056-010-1040-6] [PMID: 21082306]

[2]   Miethke RR, Brauner K. A Comparison of the periodontal health of patients during treatment with the Invisalign system and with fixed lingual appliances. J Orofac Orthop 2007; 68(3): 223-31.
[http://dx.doi.org/10.1007/s00056-007-0655-8] [PMID: 17522806]

[3]   Miller KB, McGorray SP, Womack R, *et al.* A comparison of treatment impacts between Invisalign aligner and fixed appliance therapy during the first week of treatment. Am J Orthod Dentofacial Orthop 2007; 131(3): 302.e1-9.

CHAPTER 5

Orthodontic Biomechanics Using Clear Aligners

Abstract: Orthodontic biomechanics is the foundation of orthodontic treatment. It is extremely important to fully understand orthodontic biomechanics before the clinician /orthodontist may utilize specific orthodontic appliance. This chapter highlights basic principles of biomechanics of tooth movement with emphasis on forces, moment, moment to force ratio and its importance in achieving different types of tooth movement. Also, this chapter provides detailed explanation of different types of tooth movement and relativity of moment to force ratio as well as center of rotation approximate location in each type of tooth movement. The application of these concepts with clear aligners is somehow different from the way fixed orthodontic appliance has been used. Explanation of these differences is presented.

Keywords: Aligners, Attachments, Biomechanics, Bodily, Force, Moment, Orthodontics, Ratio, Tipping, Tooth movement, Torque.

FORCE

Force is an act that when applied upon an object can change the object's state from not moving to moving and also can accelerate or decelerate moving object. Force is a vector not a scalar. This means that in order to define a force, it is important to define/describe its magnitude and direction as well as its sense. Direction is described with reference to coordinate system, in other words vertical, horizontal (medio-lateral) or front to back for example. One may call each axis, X, Y or Z for example. Sense is described in terms of right or left (In the horizontal axis), front or back (In the antero-posterior), up or down (In the vertical axis) for example. Forces may be added (if applied in the same direction and sense) or counteract each other (if applied in the same axis but in different senses/directions).

Tarek El-Bialy, Donna Galante & Sam Daher

MOMENT AND THE CONCEPT OF MOMENT TO FORCE RATIO

The concept of moment to force ratio was first introduced by Tanne *et al.*, in 1988 to define different types of tooth movement and changes of center of rotation according to changes of the moment to force ratio [1]. In short, the concept was described as follows. In order to move tooth bodily, a force must be applied to the center of mass or center of resistance of that body. In the case of teeth, the center of resistance is located somewhere in the root(s) and it is not practical to apply forces to the teeth roots.

When a force is applied to the tooth crown, usually it creates a moment (tendency for the tooth to rotate around the center of resistance) as the point of application of the force is away from the center of resistance (usually is located in the tooth root somewhere between the alveolar bone crest and tooth root apex). The produced moment is the resultant of multiplication of the magnitude of the force times the perpendicular distance from the line of action (not the point of application) of the force to the center of resistance (Fig. **5.1**).

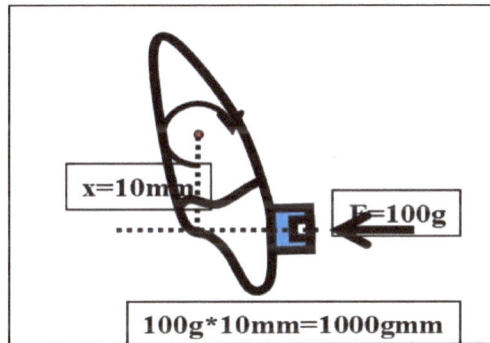

Fig. (5.1). Moment is created when a force is applied to a body (tooth in this example) away from the center of resistance. Moment = Force (100 gm) * perpendicular distance from the force line of action (dashed horizontal line) to the center of resistance (10 mm) = 1000 g mm.

In order to move a tooth bodily without applying forces to the tooth center of resistance directly that is located in the tooth root, it is important to prevent or counter act the initial moment occurred due to the applied force to the teeth crowns. To do so, a counter moment is required to negate the initial moment due to the force. *The ratio between the applied moment and the force is called moment to force ratio and this* ratio determines the resultant tooth movement (uncontrolled tipping, controlled tipping, bodily or root movement [torque]). These types of tooth movements are explained in detail below. In short, if we assume that the force will move the tooth crown tip in one direction, the counter moment would tend to move the root apex in the same direction or at least prevent the apex from movement in the opposite direction to where the tooth crown is moving.

POSSIBLE ORTHODONTIC TEETH MOVEMENT USING CLEAR ALIGNERS

Initially when clear aligners were introduced, they were introduced to solve minimum crowded teeth (1-2 mm of arch length deficiency); minimum (1-2 mm) dental spacing cases or relapsed cases.

Although many practitioners would argue that simple crowded or spacing cases can be easily corrected using routine removable or fixed orthodontic appliances, challenges as mentioned above with regular fixed appliances are cleaning, diet restriction and bracket positioning errors. Also, regular/tra-ditional removable orthodontic appliances have their own limitations which include bulkiness of the acrylic base, one point contact of the active components (wires/clasps) with the teeth which makes it difficult to control tooth movement or achieving controlled tipping or bodily movement according to the treatment goals.

In this regard, clear aligners may provide better control of tooth movement compared to traditional removable orthodontic appliances and also, when treatment planning is well-designed, difficult tooth movement including but not limited to bodily movement can be achieved.

TYPES OF ORTHODONTIC TOOTH MOVEMENTS

There are four common types of orthodontic tooth movements with regards to crown cusp tip/incisal edge -root apex relationship. There are four common types of tooth movement with regards to general body axes (vertical [intrusion/extr-usion], horizontal [buccal/lingual] and anteroposterior [proclination/retro-clination]) and with regards to the tooth own axis (rotational tooth movement).

A. **Types of Orthodontic Tooth Movements with Regards to Crown Tip-root Apex Relationship**

    a. ***Uncontrolled Tipping*** Where the tooth crown moves in one direction, while the root apex of the same tooth moves in the opposite direction (Fig. **5.2**). Normally, this type of tooth movement is produced by removable appliances using round wires, or even fixed appliances when round wires are used as the main tooth guided tooth movement. The moment to force ratio in this type of tooth movement is less than 8. Main problem with this type of tooth movement occurs when the crown moves (>1 mm) as the involved tooth root apex moves into cortical plates of bone or even out of the alveolar bone, which is usually associated with severe root resorption and/or periodontal bone defects [2 - 4]. An example of these problems can be seen in (Fig. **5.3**).

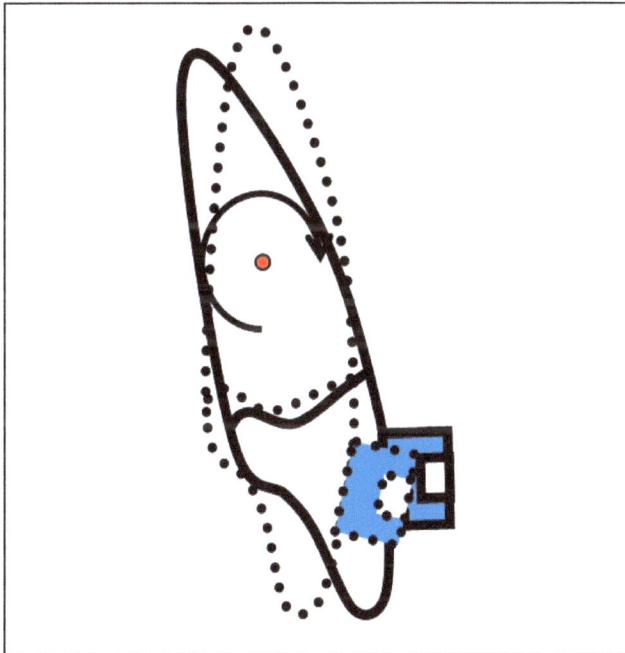

Fig. (5.2). Uncontrolled tooth movement where the tooth crown tip moves in one direction, while the tooth root apex moves in the opposite direction. Center of rotation is between center of resistance and the root apex.

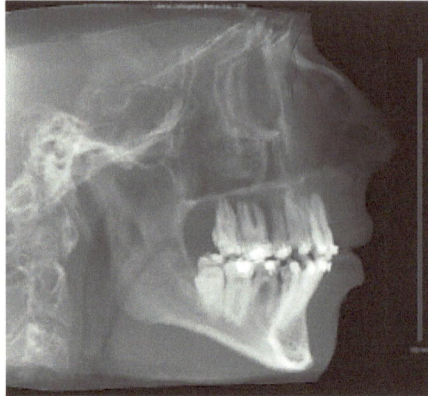

Fig. (5.3). An example of outcome of uncontrolled tooth movement where the upper central incisor's root apex moved outside the labial cortical plate of bone with high likelihood of periodontal problems like dehiscence and /or fenestration as well as root resorption.

b. ***Controlled Tipping*** Where the crown tip of a tooth moves in one direction, while the root apex of that tooth stays in the original position (Fig. **5.4**). This is called controlled because unwanted effect of the toot apex movement does not occur or less likely to occur. Usually this type of tooth movement requires application of external moment to counter act the moment due to the initial force intended to move the tooth/teeth. The moment to force ratio is around 8, depending on the tooth root length and morphology as well as level of alveolar bone.

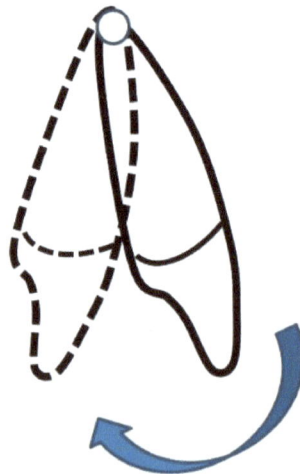

Fig. (5.4). Controlled tipping tooth movement. The center of rotation is around the tooth apex.

c. ***Bodily Movement*** In this type of tooth movement, the moment of force ratio is around 10, depending on the tooth root length, morphology and level of alveolar bone. The center of resistance would be at infinity as the assumption is that the crown and root move the same distance with almost no rotation (Fig. **5.5**).

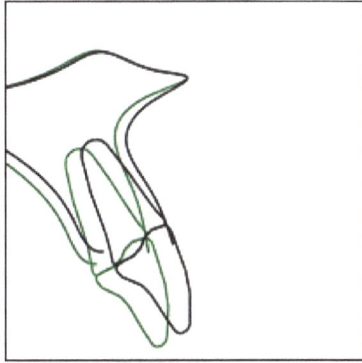

Fig. (5.5). Superimposition of cephalomteric tracing before (black) and after (green) treatment shows that the crown of the upper incisors and the root moved the same amount. Center of rotation would be in infinity.

d. ***Root Movement (Torque)*** In this type of tooth movement, the tooth root would move in one direction while the crown does not move. Moment to force ratio would be 13 or more depending on the tooth root length, morphology and level of alveolar bone crest. Center of rotation would be located around the tooth crown tip (incisal edge for example) (Fig. **5.6**).

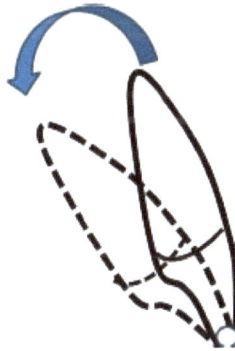

Fig. (5.6). Root movement where the root apex moves while the crown tip does not. Center of rotation would be around the incisal tip.

B. Types of Tooth Movement with Regards to General Body Axes (Vertical [Intrusion/Extrusion], Horizontal [Rbuccal/Lingual] and Anteroposterior [Proclination/Retroclination])

a. ***Intrusion/Extrusion*** Although achievable, intrusion is always produced as relative intrusion. For example, when an attempt to level curve of Spee, slight intrusion of lower incisors with proclination and premolar extrusion would achieve this goal of leveling curve of Spee. Incisor proclination (tipping crowns labially) is the easiest type of tooth movement that can be achieved by clear aligners. On the other hand, extrusion, although seems easy to be achieved by clear aligners as to provide space in the aligners for spontaneous eruption of the intended tooth or using special types of attachments/aligners configuration, it is sometimes very difficult to achieve. Simply, once an intention to extrude a tooth from labial surface, a moment is initiated that tends to move the tooth crown lingually and the tooth root labially, which in most cases, would lead to movement of the roots into labial plate of bone (cortical bone) which usually takes longer time to remodel [5]. Also, extrusion of small teeth like upper lateral or lower incisors, is somewhat challenging to be grasped by the aligners' plastics and the planned orthodontic tooth movement may be difficult to achieve. The attachments proposed by align technology that can produce extrusion are the beveled attachments [6]. The active surface is the gingivally beveled surface where the aligners' plastics apply the required extrusion forces on the teeth to be extruded (Fig. **5.7**). Intrusion normally does not require attachments on the teeth to be intruded, however anchorage teeth (lower premolars for example in case of intruding lower incisors) need to be fitted with horizontal rectangular attachments for anchorage and relative extrusion of these premolars as well.

b. ***Proclination/Reteroclination*** Anteroposterior teeth movement by clear aligners is not difficult when we consider tipping of the crowns. However, it would seem challenging moving the incisors by bodily movement. More description about possible tooth movement by clear aligners will be explained in cases in the following sections, particularly in class II cases chapter.

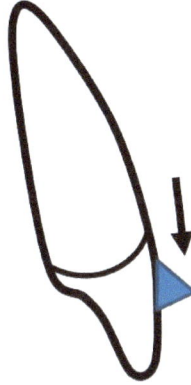

Fig. (5.7). Extrusion attachment showing the active surface and direction of extrusion forces (arrow).

c. ***Bucco-lingual Tooth Movement*** Moving posterior teeth buccally or lingually using clear aligners is not challenging as long as there is a clear freeway space or inter-occlusal clearance that allows the posterior teeth to move bucco-lingually. In order to achieve this buccolingual movement, one should consider the vertical overlap of these teeth. In other words, if the tooth intended to be moved lingually or buccally is overerupted beyond the occlusal plane, like in cases of buccal cross bite, it would be more difficult to move such a tooth buccally or lingually as it would require to have more inter-occlusal clearance than the freeway space, which is not possible or not comfortable for the patients sometimes. One option to overcome this issue is to initially intrude such an over erupted tooth then move it bucco-lingually which would complicate or make the tooth movement very time consuming.

Possible Methods of Producing Torque using Clear Aligners

An example of producing torque using clear aligner is to use what is explained by Dahr and Align technology as power ridges [4]. Power ridges together with pressure points lingually were reported to improve incisor axial inclination while retracting upper incisors to maintain torque [4]. It is assumed that power ridges would apply a lingual or palatal force on the tooth crown cervical part, which when resisted by the plastic covering the incisal edge of the same tooth creates a couple, this couple is presumed to produce lingual root torque. Although this is explicitly demonstrated, there is no available research data in the literature to support this assumption. Align technology introduced power ridges and pressure point in order to produce couple that can produce root movement in the bucco-lingual direction. A schematic sketch of this system is shown in (Fig. **5.8**) where the light arrow on the lingual side shows the pressure point close to the incisal edge, while the power ridge on the labial surface close to the gingival margin produces couple which is capable of producing the required moment to move the root palatally.

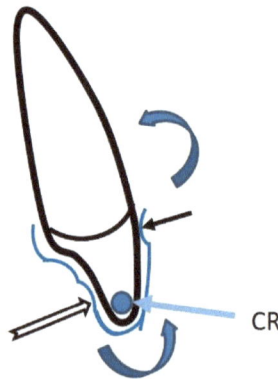

Fig. (5.8). Force system introduced by Align Technology to produce palatal root movement utilizing a couple system that is produced by a buccally and gingivally placed power ridge (Black arrow), while the other force of the couple is applied using pressure point to the lingual surface close to the incisal edge (hollow arrow). The produced moment is capable to move the roots palatally around center of rotation (CR).

A second method of producing torque is to constrain the crown position while tending to move the crown in an opposite direction to the direction of root movement. An example of what normally happens due to late mandibular forward growth or adaptation, which leads to lower incisor crowding or relapse after orthodontic treatment. In other words, if we constrain lower incisors by a fixed archwire or clear aligner and try to move upper incisors lingually while there is an adequate overbite, lingual movement of upper incisors would torque lower incisors roots labially (See Class II cases chapter).

A third possible way to torque roots with clear aligners is to move the crowns initially in the opposite direction of the intended direction of root torque. For example, if we need to torque upper incisors' roots palatally, we would move the crown labially first (counter moment first) and then moving the whole tooth palatally (Fig. **5.9**). This is similar to the traditional way of dealing with class II division 2 cases, where it is always recommended to procline upper incisors labially first (providing adequate torque) and then moving the upper incisors afterwards palatally.

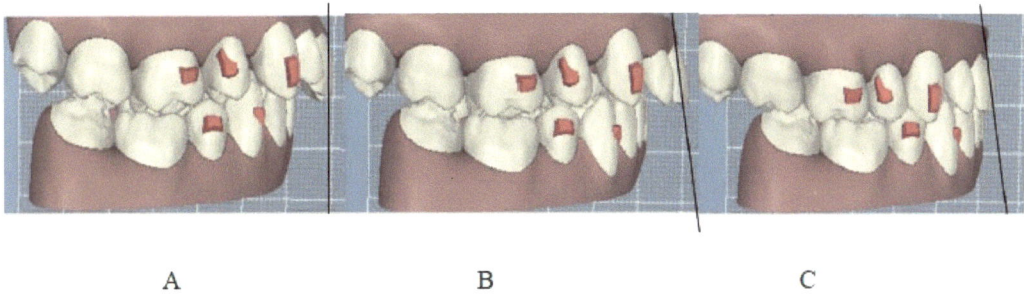

Fig. (5.9). A) initial tooth position; B) tipping upper incisors labially first (Counter moment); and then C) moving the incisors bodily palatally.

d. *Rotational Tooth Movement*

It has been reported that rotation is very challenging tooth movement with aligners [7 - 9]. However, Align technology, in their description of the optimized attachments for rotation [6], showed that these attachments have different shapes depending on the direction of the required force to rotate the involved tooth (Fig. **5.10**) [6].

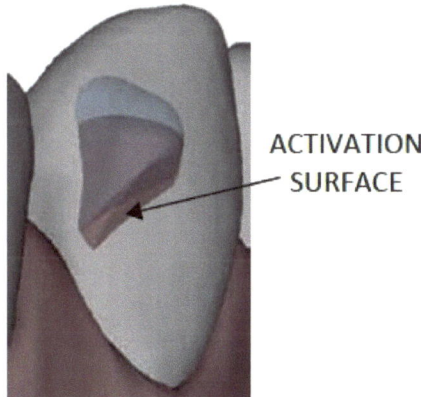

Fig. (5.10). Rotational optimized attachments as described by Align Technology [6].

e. ***Mesiodistal Root Movement Optimized Attachment*** Align technology also introduced mesiodistal root movement attachments that produce couple as described by Align Technology (Fig. **5.11**) below. The active surface on each attachment is pushed by the aligners to produce the necessary couple needed to move the teeth roots mesiodistally.

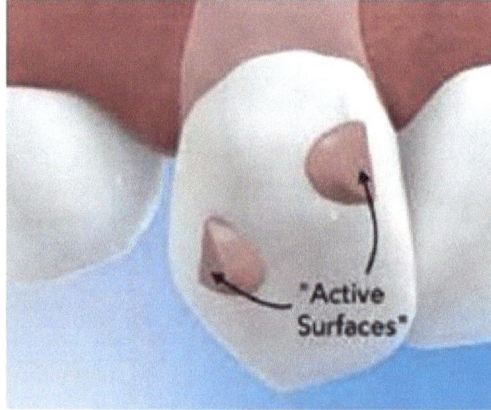

Fig. (5.11). Optimized attachments for mesiodistal root movement (Align technology) [6].

Another feature that Align Technology introduced recently is the use of precision cuts in order to support special types of tooth movements for example molar distalization. It has been recommended to use class II elastics on precision cuts on the upper canines and lower molars when distalizing upper molars to correct class II molar relationship. The reverse is also valid for class III correction. These precision cuts are meant to either apply the elastic forces directly to the aligners or to buttons bonded to teeth. More detail about these cuts and their mechanics is explained in class II and class III correction chapters later.

REFERENCES

[1]   Tanne K, Koenig HA, Burstone CJ. Moment to force ratios and the center of rotation. Am J Orthod Dentofacial Orthop 1988; 94(5): 426-31.
[http://dx.doi.org/10.1016/0889-5406(88)90133-3] [PMID: 3189245]

[2]   Mulie RM, Hoeve AT. The limitations of tooth movement within the symphysis, studied with laminagraphy and standardized occlusal films. J Clin Orthod. 1976; 12: pp. (10)882-93-6-9.

[3]   Ten Hoeve A, Mulie RM. The effect of antero-postero incisor repositioning on the palatal cortex as studied with laminagraphy. J Clin Orthod 1976; 10(11): 804-822, 886-889.
[PMID: 1069732]

[4]   Dahr S. Dr Sam Daher's Techniques for Class II Correction with Invisalign and Elastics Clinical tips and techniques by Align technology. 2011.

[5]   Turatti G, Womack R, Bracco P. Incisor intrusion with Invisalign treatment of an adult periodontal patient. J Clin Orthod 2006; 40(3): 171-4.
[PMID: 16636425]

[6]   Align technology: ATTACHMENT PROTOCOL SUMMARY online. Available at: www.aligntechinstitute.com/.../Documents/pdf/attachment_protocol.pdf

[7]   Lagravère MO, Flores-Mir C. The treatment effects of Invisalign orthodontic aligners: a systematic review. J Am Dent Assoc 2005; 136(12): 1724-9.
[http://dx.doi.org/10.14219/jada.archive.2005.0117] [PMID: 16383056]

[8]   Kravitz ND, Kusnoto B, BeGole E, Obrez A, Agran B. How well does Invisalign work? A prospective clinical study evaluating the efficacy of tooth movement with Invisalign. Am J Orthod Dentofacial Orthop 2009; 135(1): 27-35.
[http://dx.doi.org/10.1016/j.ajodo.2007.05.018] [PMID: 19121497]

[9]   Simon M, Keilig L, Schwarze J, Jung BA, Bourauel C. Treatment outcome and efficacy of an aligner technique--regarding incisor torque, premolar derotation and molar distalization. BMC Oral Health 2014; 14(68): 68.
[http://dx.doi.org/10.1186/1472-6831-14-68] [PMID: 24923279]

CHAPTER 6

Moderate and Severe Crowding Class I Cases

Abstract: Traditional approaches for treating severe crowded cases usually involve removal of some teeth with the intention to allow stable occlusion after the orthodontic treatment. However, in severe constricted cases, arch expansion could be the best approach to treat these cases without removal of permanent teeth. This chapter presents cases with severe teeth crowding and the possible treatment of these cases with clear aligners. This chapter presents moderate to severe crowding cases treated solely by clear aligners utilizing dental arch expansion. Also, this chapter presents diagnostic criteria for deciding expansion/non extraction or extraction approaches in detail.

Keywords: Class I, Expansion, Extraction, Interproximal, Malocclusion, Moderate crowding, Proclination, Severe crowding, Stripping, Spacing.

INTRODUCTION

According to Proffit [1], moderate crowding can be considered when 2-4 mm of dental arch length discrepancy exists [1]. Cases with moderate dental crowding can be treated by different approaches including expansion, proclination in cases with reteroclined upper and /or lower incisors, interproximal reduction (IPR) or extraction in cases with severe skeletal problems like increased vertical dimension/hyperdivergent or open bite cases.

The first report about treatment of moderate crowded cases by Invisalign clear aligners was reported by Boyd, in 2000 [2]. Since then, there have been many reports about the possibility of using Invisalign or clear aligners in general to treat cases with moderate crowded teeth with variable degrees of success and satisfactory finishing [3]. In addition, Boyd has introduced a new protocol for managing complex cases with Invisalign or clear aligners [4]. The following cases with moderate dental crowding were treated solely by Invisalign clear aligners,

Tarek El-Bialy, Donna Galante & Sam Daher

details are as follows.

Case 1

This twelve-year old female presented to the clinic in June 2011 with chief complaint that upper right canine tooth is labially erupted with no room/space in the dental arch to accommodate its normal position (Fig. **6.1**). The patient had relatively normal skeletal relationship, class I molars and canine relationships, upper crowding (4 mm), lower 1.5 mm crowding and upper and lower midlines coincident with facial midline.

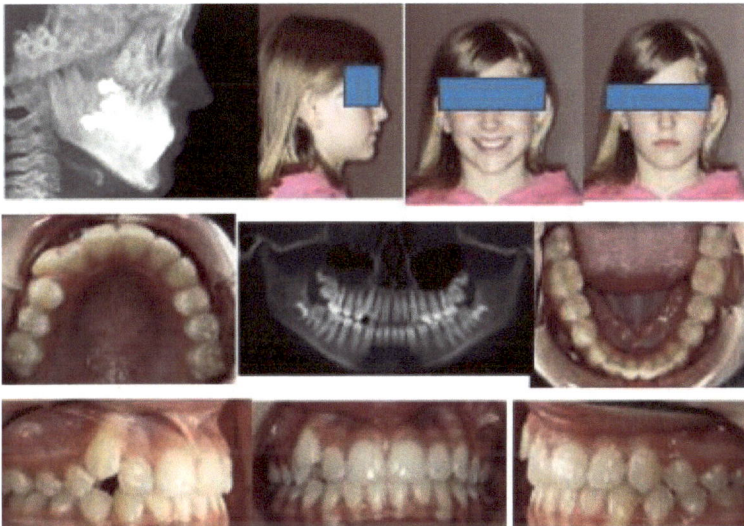

Fig. (6.1). Initial photographs of a twelve-year old female with labially erupted upper right canine tooth with upper 4 mm crowding and lower 1.5 mm crowding. Midlines are centered, right and left molars and canines are class I relationship. No Bolton discrepancy existed.

Problem List/Findings

1. Labially erupted upper right canine (4 mm crowding)
2. Slight lingually inclined upper and lower incisors
3. Right side premolars are not fully interdigitated (Slight end to end relationship) can be seen in clincheck (Fig. **6.2**).

Treatment Objectives

1. Resolve upper and lower crowding

2. Maintain midline relationships

3. Maintain left buccal occlusion and improve right occlusion.

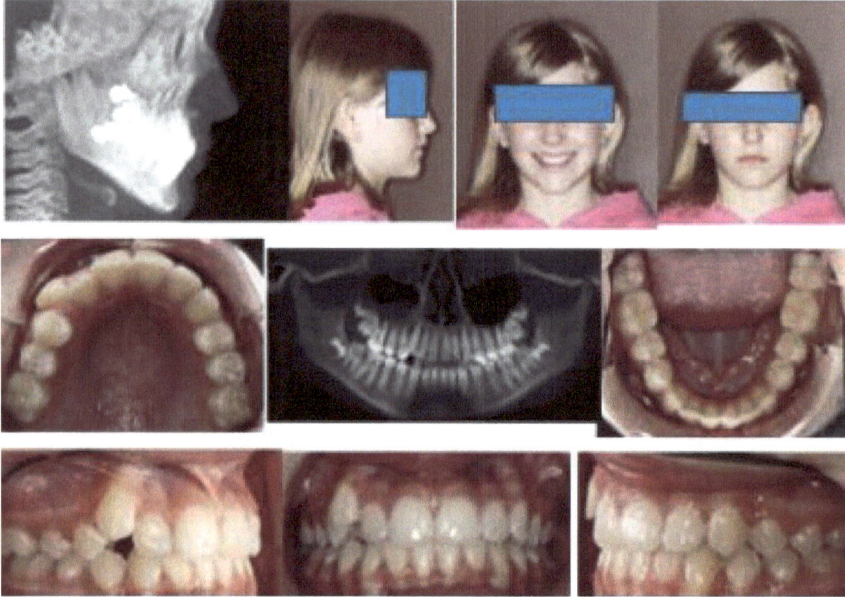

Fig. (6.2). Right side premolars are in slight end-to-end relation, and upper right first molar is not fully sucked in (full interdigitation).

Treatment plan included sight expansion (non-extraction) of the upper and lower arches and labial crown torque of upper incisors.

Two treatment options were presented to the patient:

1. Full fixed appliance, or

2. Invisalign clear aligners treatment

Parents and patient were informed with limitations of each technique and both patient and parents chose Invisalign treatment. Patient was fitted with 22 aligners, utilizing class II elastics on both sides to improve buccal occlusion, providing space for upper right canine and left class II elastics were used to prevent canting of anterior occlusal plan. Also, slight proclination of the upper and lower incisors were requested 1) improve their position, and 2) provide space for the buccally erupted upper right canine. (Fig. **6.3**): shows patient after 11 months in treatment with no refinement or second set of aligners. Fig. (**6.4**) shows superimposition of initial and final tooth position as produced by Clincheck®. It can be observed that the upper right canine moved favorably into its normal position, while midlines were maintained, buccal occlusions were improved to full class I molars and premolars.

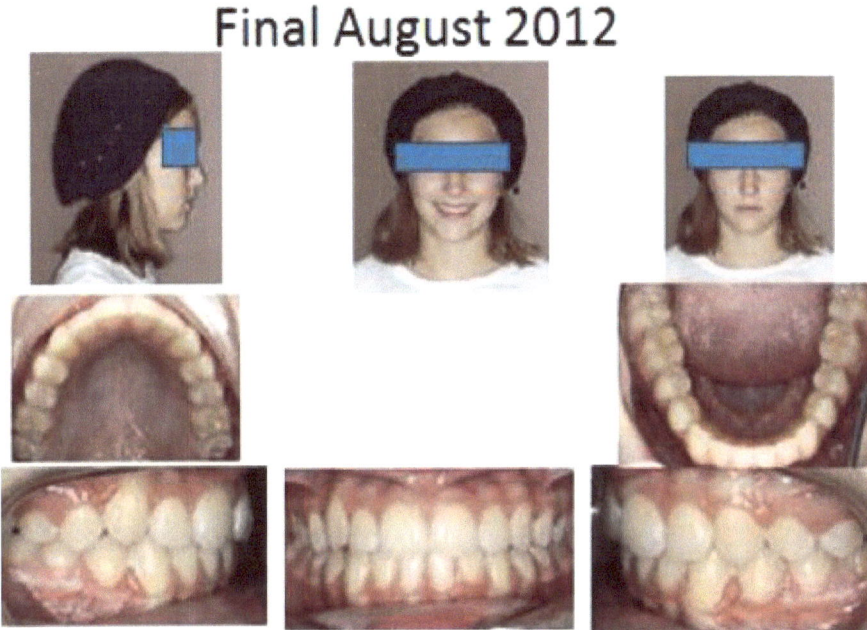

Fig. (**6.3**). Final photos after one year in treatment.

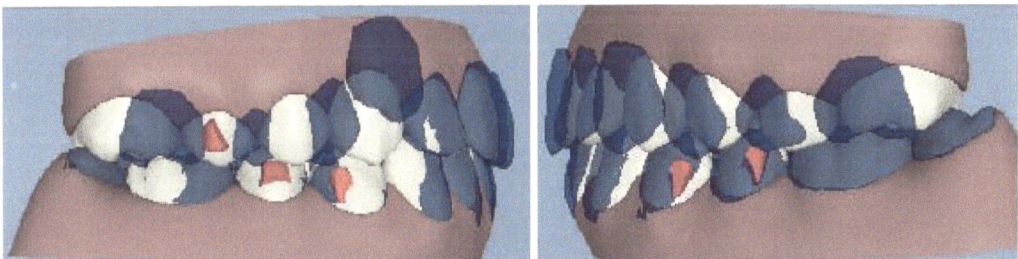

Fig. (**6.4**). Model superimposition showing initial position (blue) and final toot position (white).

Retention protocol includes 24/7 earing of Vivera upper and lower retainers in the first year and night time afterwards (forever). Possible relapse without wearing retainers was explained possibly due to normal growth or facial adaptation.

Severe Crowding Cases

Severe crowding according to Proffit is defined as arch length deficiency of more than 3 mm [5]. In this regard, the case presented above may be considered severe crowding as well. The next case is definitely severe crowding and traditional orthodontic treatment plan is recommended for doing serial extraction. It has been reported that the use of lingual arch in late mixed dentition can be helpful in resolving incisor crowding [6, 7]. The idea of using lingual arch in late mixed dentition is to save leeway space (E-Space) to resolve moderate crowding (2-4 mm).

Case 2

This 10 years old boy was referred to our clinic by his general dentist for space management due to early loss of upper right second deciduous molar and lower right deciduous canine teeth (Fig. **6.5**).

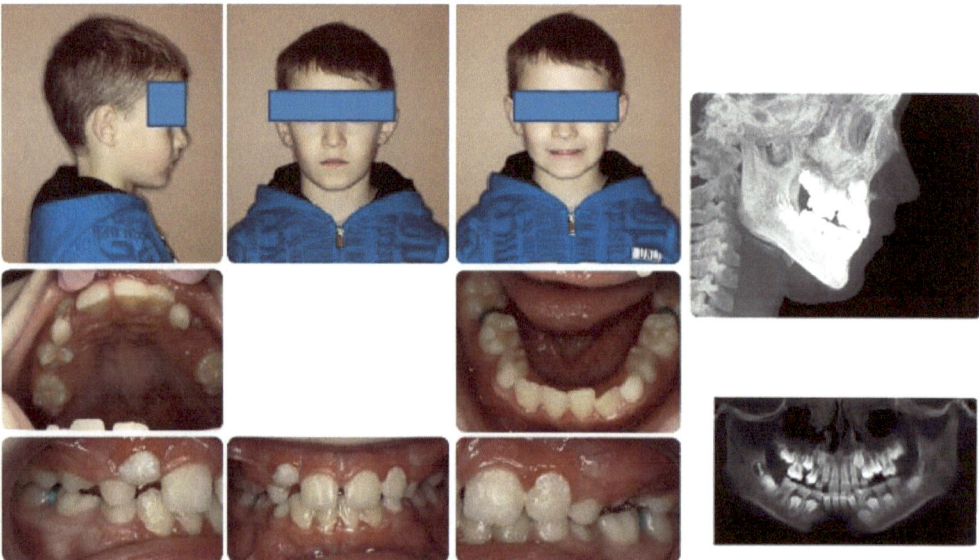

Fig. (6.5). 10 years old boy presented with severe crowding (blocked upper right second premolar and lower right canine and also crowding in the area of upper left canine/premolars area due to premature loss of upper left deciduous molars.

Treatment options that were discussed with the patient and parents included utilization of Wilson 3D space maintainers/arch expanders in an attempt to preserve/create some spaces for the erupting permanent teeth. As phase I treatment, this would not preclude an extraction treatment in phase II if there is a need to do so in the future. Other option was to wait and watch however less likely a non-extraction treatment would be a likelihood Phase II option. Patient and parents agreed to start Phase I utilizing Wilson 3D upper Quad Helix and lower active lingual arch (RMO, Denver, CO, USA) in attempt to maintain/recreate spaces for the erupting permanent premolars and canine teeth. Cephalometric analysis showed average skeletal and dental analysis that did not require specific attention or concern. Patient was fitted with Wilson 3D upper quad helix and lower active lingual arch appliances in December 2010. Active treatment and adjustments were performed over three month intervals for a year and four months. Treatment results of phase I are shown in (Fig. **6.6**).

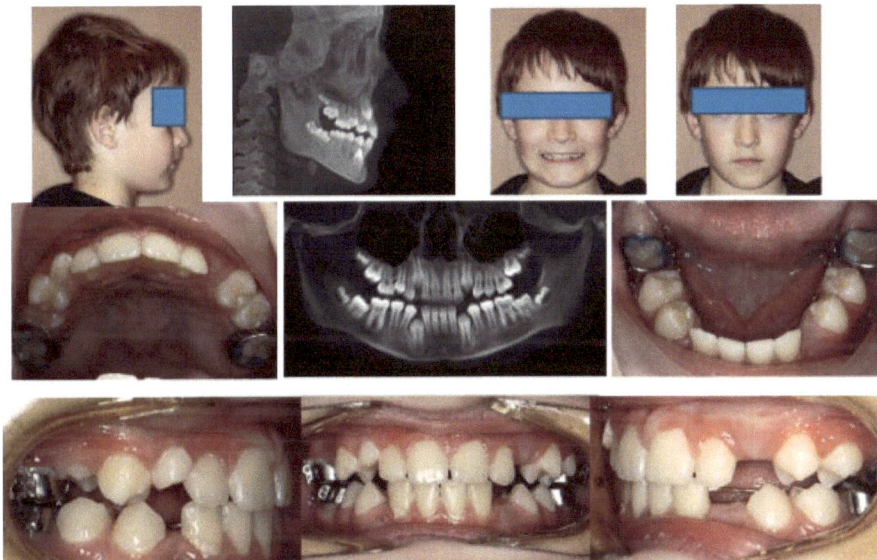

Fig. (6.6). Patient after Phase I orthodontic treatment. It can be noticed that upper right second premolar is partially erupted. First quadrant still requires at least 3 mm to fit in all premolars and canine. There is 2-3 mm of space available in the lower right quadrant, however, it still requires at least 4 mm in this quadrant to fit in the lower right permanent canine. Quadrants 2 and 3 require at least 3 mm each to fit in the erupting canines. In total, upper arch length deficiency is about 6-7 mm, and lower arch length deficiency is 6-7 mm, which makes the case challenging to be solved by non-extraction treatment plan.

Phase II was discussed with the patient and parents who both declined fixed orthodontic braces treatment and required Invisalign treatment. Patient's clincheck included 22 aligners and the plan was to expand the upper and lower arches slightly and to procline upper and lower incisors slightly as his profile allows for slight incisor proclination. Fig. (**6.7**) shows progress photos in August (4 months of Invisalign treatment) and February 2013 (10 months of treatment) which show that upper right second premolar has erupted into occlusion, upper left and lower right and left canines have erupted, and upper right canine is about to erupt. Clincheck initial (blue) and final tooth position superimposition is coincident with the clinical progress photos. Clincheck superimposition shows slight lateral expansion as well as slight AP expansion which provided enough spaces for the blocked teeth to erupt normally. A critical review of this case may criticize long-term stability of such expansion. Retention protocol in any expansion, in my opinion is night time for life after a year of full time (20-22 hours daily) retainer wear. It is important to follow up on the eruption of second and third molars.

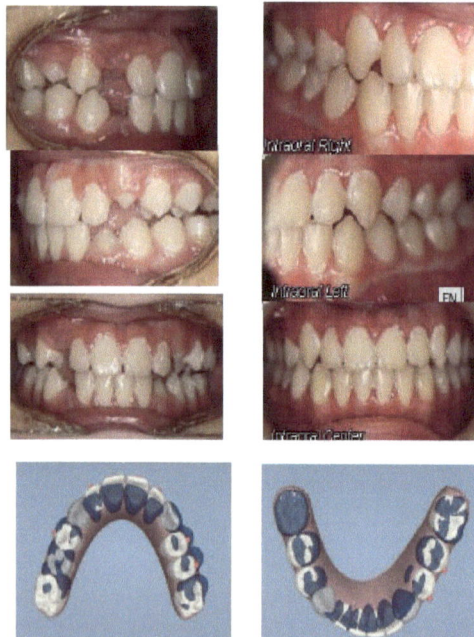

Fig. (6.7). Left column shows 2 months into Invisalign treatment photos (August 2012). It can be seen that upper and lower left canines are erupting and upper right second premolar erupted into normal occlusion. Right column shows progress photos in May 2013 which show upper and lower left canines erupted into full occlusion. Also, lower right canine that was initially blocked due to no space for it, is now erupting. Space for upper right canine is provided and this canine is about to erupt.

Case 3

This is a 47 years old female who presented to the clinic with chief complaint of large spaces between the front teeth. She wanted to improve/close these spaces whenever possible. Clinical records (Fig. **6.8**) show that she has a convex profile with slightly increased nasolabial angle and recessive chin. She was not concerned about her convex profile but mainly concerned about spacing between her front teeth. Intraoral examination revealed class I molars and canine relationships. Acceptably positioned upper incisors and proclined lower incisors and upper dental arch spacing (7 mm) and lower arch spacing (5 mm). Cephalometric analysis (Table **1**) revealed class II skeletal relationship due to prognathic maxilla, which is acceptable for her ethnic background. Also, cephalometric analysis revealed that upper incisors were retroclined to acceptable and lower incisors were proclined (compensating for the skeletal Class II relationship).

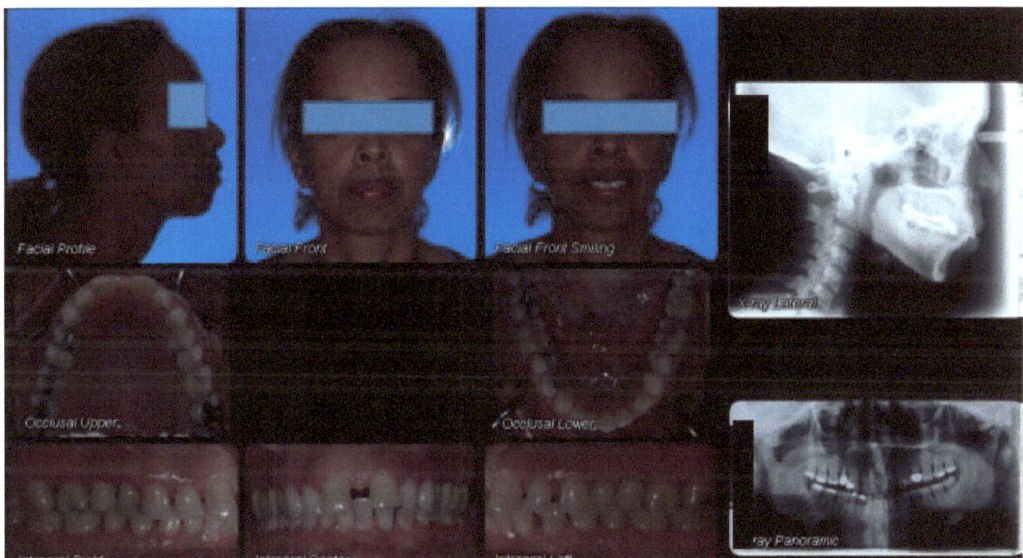

Fig. (6.8). Clinical records before treatment show convex profile with recessive chin, hypermentalis muscle activity and upper and lower severe spacing. Bolton analysis revealed increased lower anterior ratio by 1.5 mm due to small upper lateral incisors.

Although this is a skeletal class II case, which could have been discussed in Chapter 8 (Class II cases), I preferred to discuss this case here in class I malocclusion chapter as the patient's desire was not to change her profile and accept the skeletal relationship. Also, dental occlusion of this case is class I buccal relationship; which makes the case suitable to be discussed here in class I cases chapter. As the patient declined surgical option to fix her skeletal relationship, we were left with only one option which is camouflage treatment. Treatment objectives were to maintain skeletal relationship, close upper and lower spaces and leave some spaces distal to upper lateral incisors build up later on. Treatment included maximum retraction of upper and lower incisors, while palatally torqueing upper incisors and maintaining posterior occlusion as it is. The patient clincheck showed 23 aligners that finished in 44 weeks. Treatment results (Fig. **6.9**, Table **1**) show improvement in lower incisor position (protrusion and retroclination) and retroclination of upper incisors. As indicated in (Fig. **6.10**) (Superimposition), maximum retraction of upper and lower incisors was achieved while posterior occlusion was maintained.

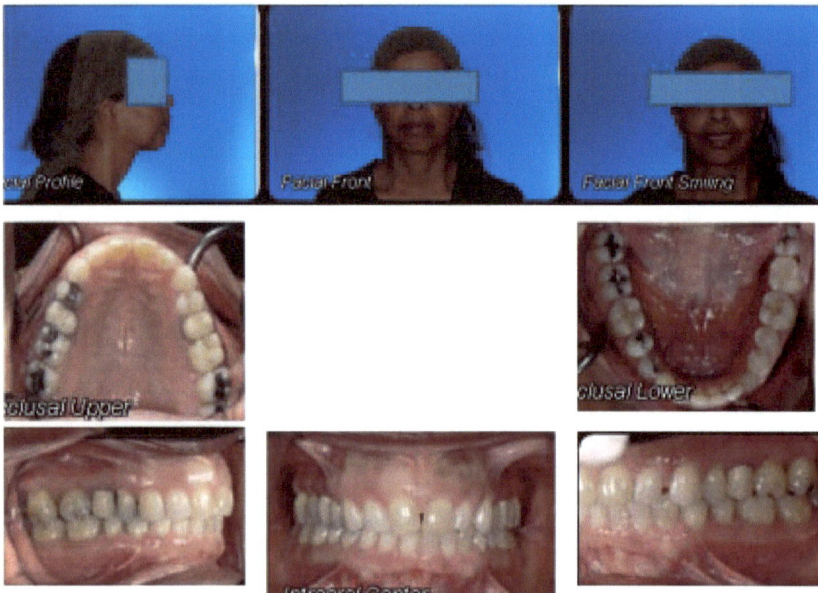

Fig. (6.9). Clinical records after treatment showing consolidating of the spaces while minor spacing was left distal to upper left lateral incisor for buildup. Also, 0.5 mm median diastema was left and accepted by the patient.

In summary, moderate or severe crowded cases may be treated successfully with clear aligners once appropriate diagnosis and treatment planning has been performed according to clear insights into each case, particularly using CBCT.

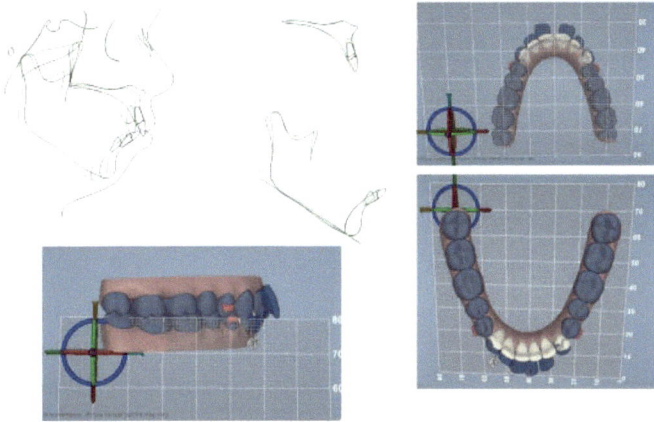

Fig. (6.10). Cephalomteric and clincheck superimpositions showing the amount of incisor retractions. Also upper and lower incisors were tipped lingually by controlled tipping type of tooth movement.

Table 1. Cephalometric analyses before and after 22 aligners (44 weeks of treatment).

		Initial	Final
Skeletal	SNA (°)	89	85.9
	SNB (°)	79.7	77.1
	ANB (°)	9.3	8.8
	Wits Appraisal (mm)	5.3	5.7
	Y-Axis -- Downs (SGn-FH) (°)	61.7	64.2
	FMA (MP-FH) (°)	25.2	29.8
	LFH/TFH (ANS-Me:N-Me) (%)	59.1	58
Dental	Interincisal Angle (U1-L1) (°)	115.5	138.7
	U1 - NA (mm)	4	-0.6
	U-Incisor Protrusion (U1-APo) (mm)	11.7	7
	U1 - NA (°)	14.4	5.6
	U1 - SN (°)	103.3	91.5
	L1 - NB (mm)	14.8	8.9
	L1 - NB (°)	40.9	26.9
	L1 - Occ Plane (°)	55.3	68.5
	IMPA (L1-MP) (°)	109.7	92.7
Soft Tissue	Lower Lip to E-Plane (mm)	8.4	3.3
	Upper Lip to E-Plane (mm)	2.4	0.8
	Nasolabial Angle (Col-Sn-UL) (°)	112.2	116.5

REFERENCES

[1]   Proffit WR, Fields HW. Contemporary Orthodontics. 5th ed. Mosby 2013; p. 247.

[2]   Boyd R, Miller RJ, Vlaskalic V. The Invisalign system in adult orthodontics: mild crowding and space closure cases. J Clin Orthod 2000; (34): 13-5.

[3]   Vlaskalic V, Boyd RL. Orthodontic treatment of a mildly crowded malocclusion using the Invisalign System. Aust Orthod J 2001; (17): 41-6.

[4]   Boyd RL. Complex Orthodontic Treatment Using a New Protocol for the Invisalign Appliance. JCO 2007; 9(XLI): 525-47.

[5]   Proffit WR, Fields HW. Contemporary Orthodontics. 5th ed. Mosby 2013; p. 477.

[6]   Brennan MM, Gianelly AA. The use of the lingual arch in the mixed dentition to resolve incisor crowding. Am J Orthod Dentofacial Orthop 2000; 117(1): 81-5.
[http://dx.doi.org/10.1016/S0889-5406(00)70252-6]

[7]   Proffit WR, Fields HW. Contemporary Orthodontics. 5th ed. Mosby 2013; p. 477.

CHAPTER 7

Treatment of Class II Malocclusion Using Clear Aligners

Abstract: Although it has been reported earlier in 2005 that it is difficult to achieve full correction of sagittal relationship (class II or III) either dental or skeletal using clear aligners, pioneer reports by Boyd and Dahr [1, 2] have been stimulating to the creativity of orthodontists who may modify original protocols that were provided by Boyed and Dahr. Proper designing clincheck or treatment planning in class II cases is very important utilizing the principles of both functional appliances and bioprogressive techniques. The following cases will explain how to utilize both functional appliance and bioprogressive principles using clear aligners to correct class II cases. Although, this might seem as case reports or case series, further clinical trials are required to support or otherwise provide other evidences of using clear aligners in correcting class II skeletal and dental cases.

Keywords: Bioprogressive, CBCT, Class II, Clear aligners, Growth modification, Growth prediction, Mechanics, Skeletal, Technique, Treatment planning.

INTRODUCTION

Previous reports have shown that class II cases can be treated by clear aligners [1 - 2]. All available publications in the literature are limited to the use of Invisalign for this type of treatment with no other clear aligners being reported to correct sagittal jaw discrepancy. Different protocols have been reported for class II treatment planning, however the most common ones are: 1) Premolar extraction using 1 mm rectangular attachments for root parallelism using Boyd protocol [1]; 2) Upper arch expansion and upper molar distalization using Dahr protocol where he proposes buccal crown torque (Power Ridge™ feature) on the upper incisors as he starts retraction on the incisors and lingual root torque on the lower incisors [2]. Also, in cases where upper molars distalization is recommended, third molars

Tarek El-Bialy, Donna Galante & Sam Daher

are recommended to be removed to allow for distalization of upper molars. In this case, class II elastics are recommended to be used to support anterior anchorage. According to Dahr [2], if buttons are to be used on the upper canines, it would be better to bond the buttons on the labial surfaces of the upper canines to apply distalization forces closer to the center of rotation.

In my opinion, center of rotation is a function of the tooth movement and it is less predictable to estimate its position, while center of resistance of the tooth is more predictable to locate. Applying the force as cervical as the crown allows, still create moment that tends to tip the canine crown distally and the root mesially by uncontrolled tooth movement. The protocol that has been recommended by Boyed seems to be valid that recommends using vertical square attachments on the canines that can provide couple, this couple can move the canine roots distally along with the crown tips. A detailed explanation of the two views is in the following sketch (Fig. **7.1**).

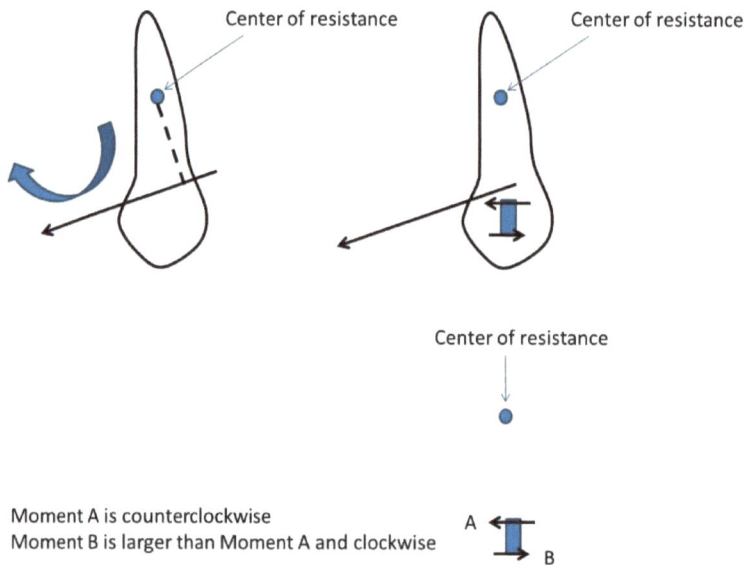

Moment A is counterclockwise
Moment B is larger than Moment A and clockwise

Fig. (7.1). Moment on upper canine without vertical attachment leads to clockwise moment and distal crown tipping of upper canine with most likely uncontrolled tipping of the canine. With vertical attachments (Right figure), a coupe is created with class II elastics that can lead to counter-clockwise moment that automatically upright the canine while retracting with class II elastics or any distal force. Detailed biomechanical analysis of vertical and optimized attachments are underway to provide the best option of either attachments for space closure.

As mentioned before in chapter 6, in order to correct class II malocclusion with proclined upper incisors, if the treatment objectives are to retract upper incisors by bodily movement, palatal root torque (labial crown tip/torque) is required to maintain proper axial inclination of upper incisors.

In his white paper, Dahr 2011 [2] presented an interesting protocol of class II correction with emphasis on using class II elastics and upper molar distalization. This chapter emphasizes on upper and lower incisor torque consideration and possible growth modification using clear aligners.

Previous case reports and publications about treatment of class II solely by Invisalign showed improvement of buccal occlusion, overbite and overjet [1 - 3]. However, most of these reports showed proclination of the lower incisors, in particular when class II elastics were used to distalize upper molars [2, 3], except cases reported by Boyed that showed lower incisor inclination is actually improved after treatment [1]. Exact mechanisms of how lower incisor inclination was improved in Boyed cases were not explicitly explained. In cases where lower incisor inclination are retroclined, it is understandable that class II elastics can procline lower incisors to normal position, however in cases with proclined lower incisors, it is unclear how mechanism(s) were used to retroclined after class II elastics. One can assume that lower crown torque or lower incisor pre-retroclination was requested/performed. This technique looks like the best way of handling class II, especially when class II elastics may be used to distalize upper molars.

Case 1: Class II With Bimaxillary Protrusion

A 19 year-old-female was presented to the clinic with a chief complaint of upper and lower front teeth sticking out that required improvement. Initial records in June 2008 revealed that the patient had a skeletal class II as seen by convex profile with retrognathic mandible and slightly recessive chin (Fig. **7.2**). Regardless of the convex profile, it was accepted by the patient and she did not want to change it. Cephalometric measurements revealed bimaxillary dentoalveolar protrusion and proclination (Fig. **7.3**), (Table **7.1**). Lower incisor inclination was planned to be retroclined (lingual crown torque). Upper incisors were requested to be retracted to close all spaces (5 mm) in the upper arch. No Class II elastics were prescribed. Clincheck is seen in (Fig. **7.4**).

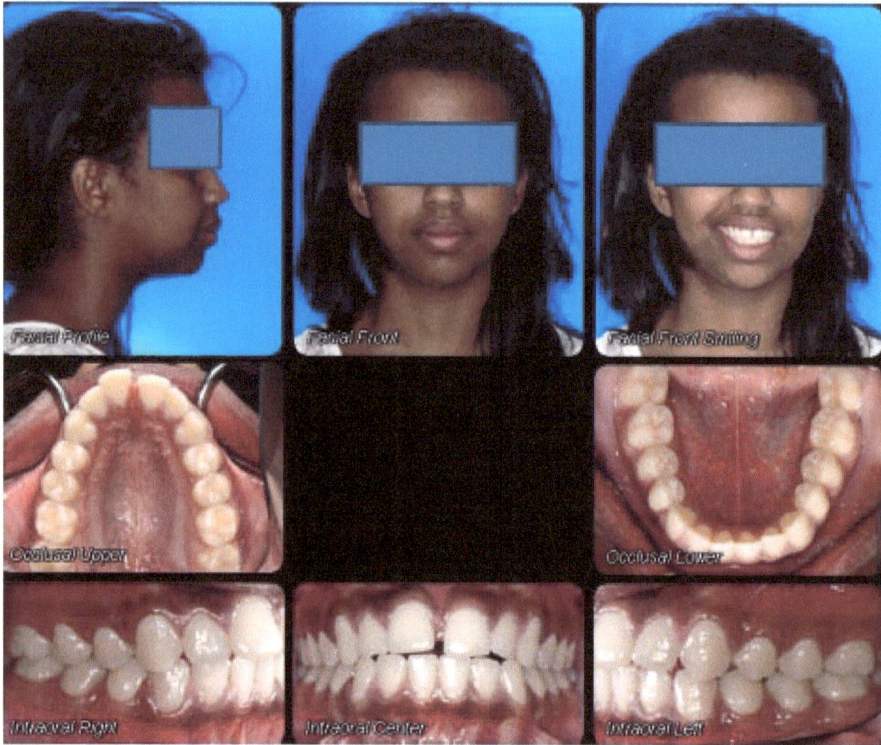

Fig. (7.2). 19 years old female with bimaxillary dental protrusion and retrognathic chin.

Table 7.1. Cephalometric analysis before and after treatment.

		Initial	Final
Skeletal	SNA (°)	85.8	85.1
	SNB (°)	79.3	78.5
	ANB (°)	6.4	6.4
	Wits Appraisal (mm)	3.6	3.3
	FMA (MP-FH) (°)	28.5	28.9
	Lower Face Height (ANS-Me) (mm)	63.8	61.8
	N-Me (mm)	111.7	110.1
	Y-Axis -- Downs (SGn-FH) (°)	59.6	57.9

(Table 7.1) contd.....

		Initial	Final
Dental	Interincisal Angle (U1-L1) (°)	103.8	117.9
	U1 - NA (mm)	8.9	5.7
	U-Incisor Protrusion (U1-APo) (mm)	13.6	10.4
	U1 - NA (°)	31.4	24.6
	U1 - SN (°)	117.2	109.7
	L1 - NB (mm)	10.9	9.7
	L1 - NB (°)	38.4	31
	IMPA (L1-MP) (°)	98.8	90.6
Soft Tissue	Lower Lip to E-Plane (mm)	4.8	5.7
	Upper Lip to E-Plane (mm)	0.6	1.4
	Nasolabial Angle (Col-Sn-UL) (°)	99.3	93.1
	Facial Convexity (G'-Sn-Po') (°)	19.7	22
	Upper Lip to Incisor (UL-U1) (mm)	1.4	2.2

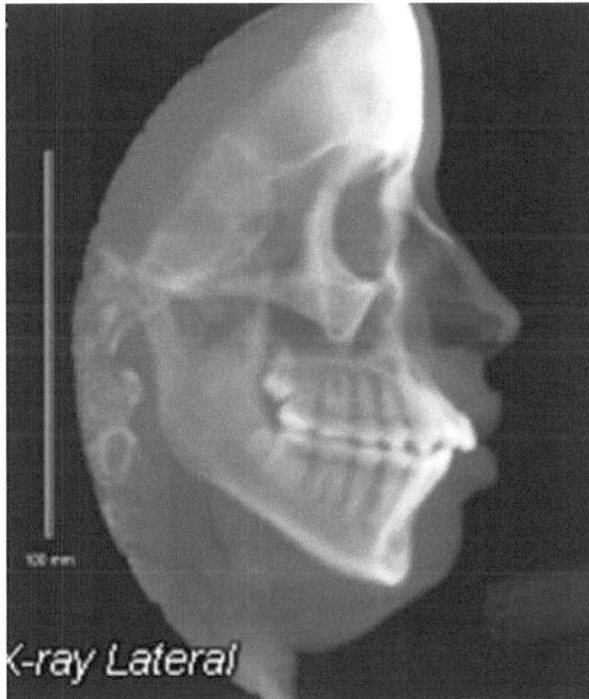

Fig. (7.3). Initial cephalometric radiographs showing bimaxillary protrusion.

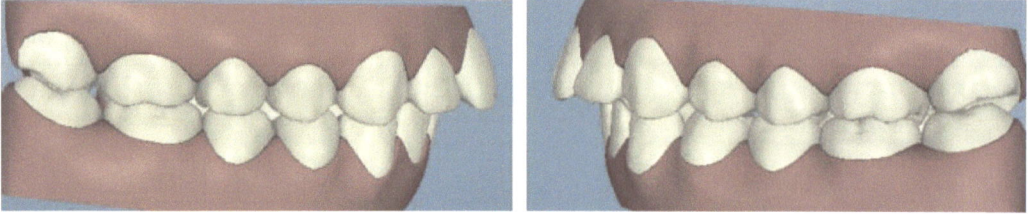

Fig. (7.4). Clincheck side view, show class II end to end relationship of the right and left buccal segments.

Results

Fig. (**7.5**) shows that Class II correction was achieved mainly by upper molar de-rotation. Since upper incisor retraction was more than the lower incisor retraction, the achieved labial root torque is assumed to be due to lingual crown torque of the lower incisors by retraction of upper incisors more than the lower (Figs. **7.6** and **7.7**, Table **7.1**), however due to the resultant overbite, upper incisors did not go to cross bite and instead, upper incisors' retraction produced lower incisor lingual crown (labial root) torque. Upper and lower incisors' inclination and protrusion were improved mainly by retraction and closing by upper and lower spaces.

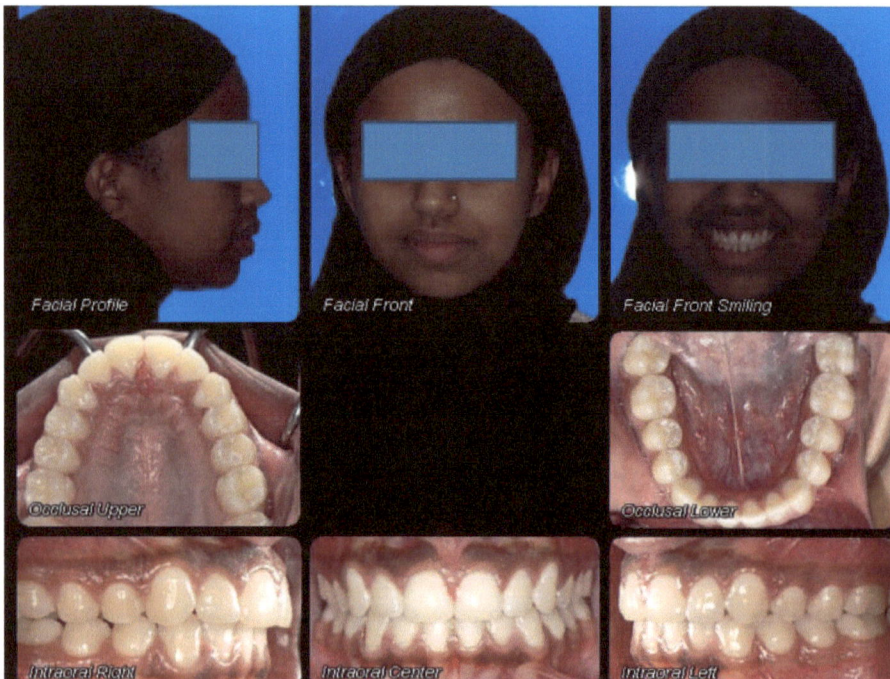

Fig. (7.5). Clinical photos of the Patient AB19 after treatment.

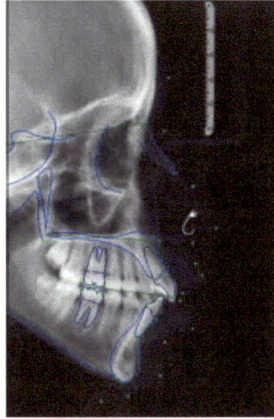

Fig. (7.6). Cephalometric radiograph for Patient AB 19 after treatment.

Although FMA did not change much, Y-axis was closed and this could be attributed to the fact that the occlusal covering of posterior teeth might have been working as a posterior bite blocks that led to slight intrusion of posterior teeth and consequently slight autorotation of the mandible, improving class II as well as Y-axis and recessive chin.

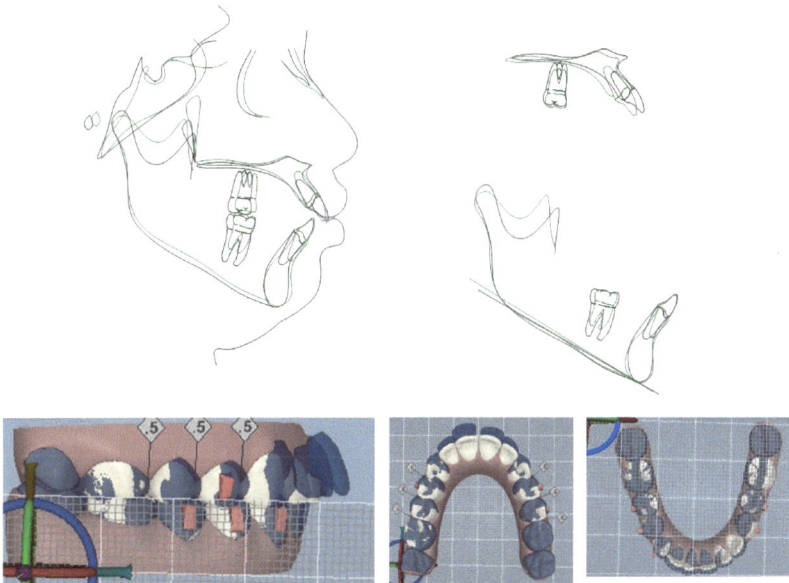

Fig. (7.7). Patient AB19 superimposition of before and after treatment cephalometric digitized tracings and clincheck. Difference of incisor position before and after treatment can be seen.

Superimpositions of before and after cephalometric digitization as well as clincheck superimposition (Fig. **7.7** and Table **7.1**) show that upper incisors were retracted while lower incisors were torqued (labial root torque [lingual crown torque]). The obtained lower incisor lingual crown torque by maximum retraction of upper incisors seems to be a new and novel approach to control lower incisors' inclination. A valid criticism would be that this acheived lingual crown torque of lower incisors could be just a cephalometric tracing error that needs further documentation. The following cases are the best proof of this principle using cone-beam-computed-tomography (CBCT).

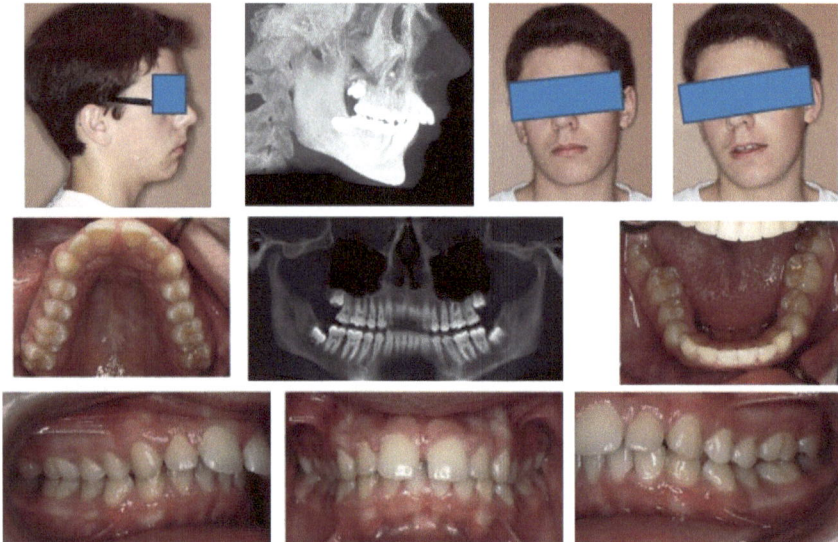

Fig. (7.8). Clinical photos and cephalometric radiographs generated from initial CBCT of patient LJ that show convex profile and recessive chin. Class II division 1 malocclusion with impinging overbite and median diastema. Patient was biting on the plastic bite-piece while scanning CT which could show an over presented class II. However, upon autorotation of the mandible using Anatomage and re-digitization, cephalometric analysis confirm class II as outlined in figures 7.9 and 7.10 below.

Case 2: Class II

A 15 year-old male was presented to the clinic with chief complaint of sticking out and spaced upper front teeth that needed to be fixed. No medical history of concern was recognized. Clinical records showed that he has meso-cephalic facial form and convex profile due to recessive chin (Fig. **7.8**). Digital models showed a class II division 1 malocclusion with overjet 11.5 mm and 100% overbite. Mild upper spacing and minimal lower dental arch crowding (Fig. **7.9**). Cephalometric records and analysis confirmed that the patient has a skeletal class II relationship due to mandibular reterognathism, bimaxillary dentoalveolar protrusion and proclined upper and lower incisors (Fig. **7.10**, Table **7.2**). TMJ tomograms showed forward inclined mandibular condyles, which according to Bjork [4], provides the likelihood of late forward mandibular growth.

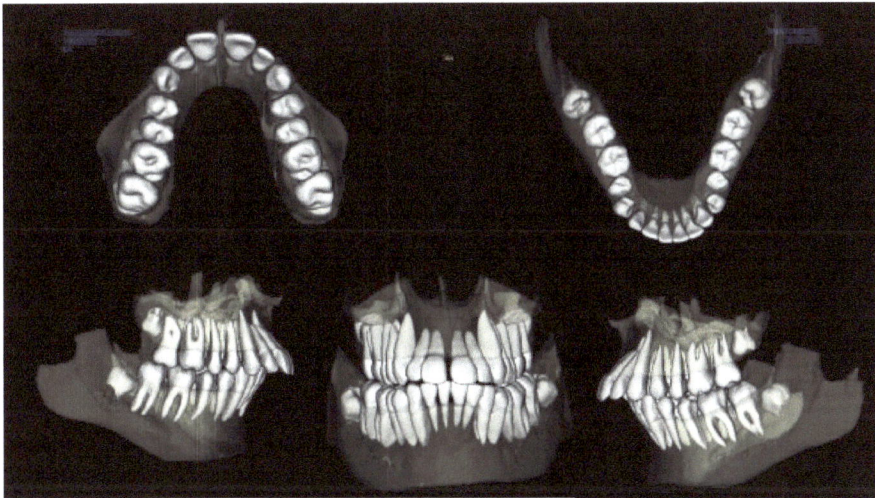

Fig. (7.9). Initial digital models show full step Class II division 1 malocclusion. Overjet is 11.3 mm.

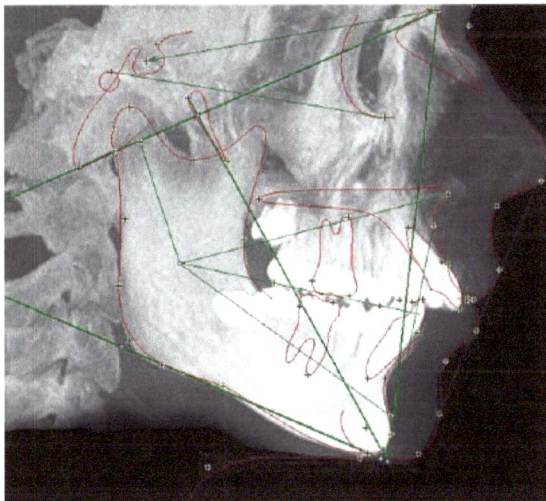

Fig. (7.10). Patient LJ Initial cephalometric radiograph and analysis. It can be seen that the patient has a skeletal class II due to mandibular reterognathism with bimaxillary dentoalveolar protrusion/proclination.

Table 7.2. Confirms class II skeletal relationship with bimaxillary dentoalveolar protrusion.

Variable	Clinical Norm	Value
NPogFH	87±3°	93°
FH to S-N	7±3°	19°
SNA	82±2°	79°
SNB	80±2°	72°
ANB	2±2°	7°
WITS	-1±1mm	8mm
NAPog	0.0±5.1°	11°
FH to Me-Go	29±4°	15°
S-N to Me-Go	36±5°	34°
S-N to Occ.	17±4°	16°
N-S-Gn	67±3°	67°
1u to SN	102±2°	115°
Max1-NA	22.0°	35.9°
1u-NA	4mm	4mm
II	130.0..150.0°	109.4°
1l to Go-Me	90±2°	103°
Mand1-NB	25.0°	27.5°
1l-NB	4mm	6mm
1l to A-Pog	1±2mm	1mm
1l to A-Pog Ang.	22±4°	24°
Pog-NB		3mm
Nasolabial Angle	110±10°	117°

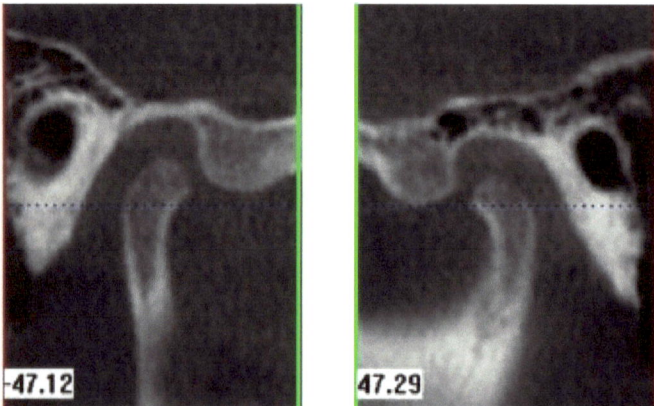

Fig. (7.11). Tomograms while the patient was biting on plastic piece for iCAT CBCT showing the condylar heads are directed forward however their position is slightly downward. It is to be noted that cephalogram, even if generated from CBCT usually do not show direction of condylar heads.

TMJ tomogram (Fig. **7.11**) shows forward direction of mandibular condyles.

Patient accepted last option and chose Invisalign treatment. The patient was referred for extraction of upper and lower third molars. However, the patient did not proceed with the extraction due to personal matters.

Treatment Planning

Patient was fitted with 52 Invisalign aligners that were programmed to achieve upper molar distalization utilizing intermaxillary class II elastics. Lower incisors' proclination was controlled by reteroclining them to counteract their possible forward proclination due to class II elastics.

Due to insufficient spaces in the lower arch, lower interproximal reduction (IPR) was requested.

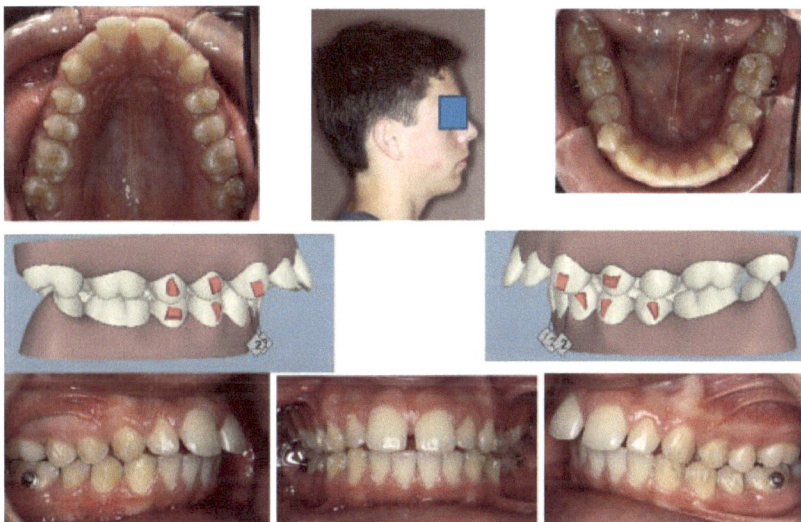

Fig. (7.12). Clincheck at stage 17 showing edge to edge molars and premolars while canines are class II, in contrast clinical photos showing interdigitized molars to canines in a full class I relationship. Also, even at stage 17/52, profile has already been improved compared to initial profile.

Treatment Progress

Patient was advised to use class II elastics (3/16" 4.5 oz.) and wear the aligners 20-22 hours/day. Also, patient was advised to change the aligners every 10 days, or whenever the trays are felt loose. At stage 17 (aligner # 17), clincheck showed an end-to-end relationship of the molars and premolars as well as class II canine relationship on both sides, while clinical photographs show full class I molars to canines (Fig. **7.12**). At stage 35, clincheck shows class I molars to canines on both sides, however clinical photos show class III tendency (Fig. **7.13**). The patient was checked clinically for any dual bite or forward shift but there was no such dual bite or forward shift noticed clinically.

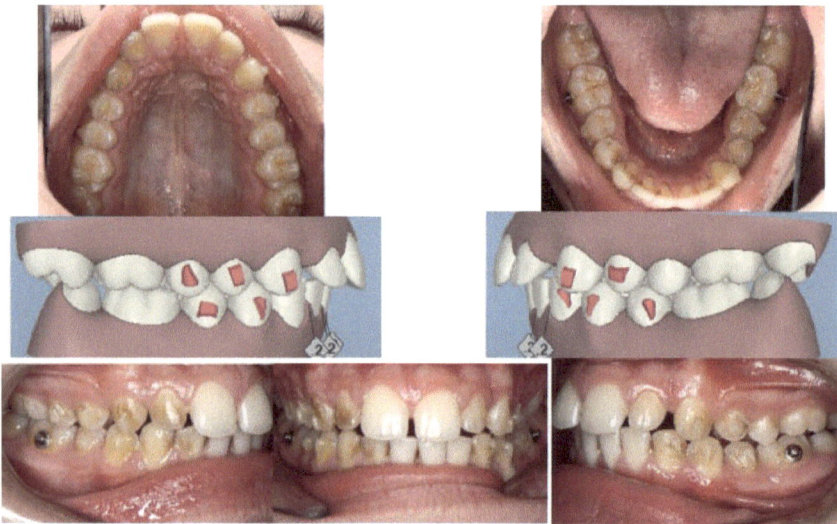

Fig. (7.13). Clincheck at stage 39 showing class I buccal segment while clinical photos showing class III tendency. Also, according to the clincheck at this stage, there should have been about 4 mm of overjet that allows for retraction of upper incisors and closing upper spaces. However, clinically, there was less than 1 mm overjet. Upper right lateral incisors are almost in edge-to-edge relationship.

Due to concern of having the patient getting into anterior cross bite (of lateral incisors), patient was instructed to stop using class II elastics at this stage. Patient was carefully seen every two weeks to manage any possible cross bite that might happen. Patient continued to were aligners to the end without elastics. After 15 months, final occlusion was excellent and the patient did not require any further aligners. Final records were obtained then and patient was fitted with Vivera retainers. Final records including cephalomteric radiographs showed improvement of the patient's facial profile (Fig. **7.14**) and cephalometric superimposition revealed mandibular forward growth (Fig. **7.15**, Table **7.3**). Forward mandibular growth explains the overcorrection of the patient's occlusion during treatment compared to the clincheck at stages 17 and 35. It is has been speculated that clear aligners might have worked as functional appliance at this stage. Fig. (**7.14**) also shows CBCT-generated tomograms of the patient showing the condyle in centric relationship.

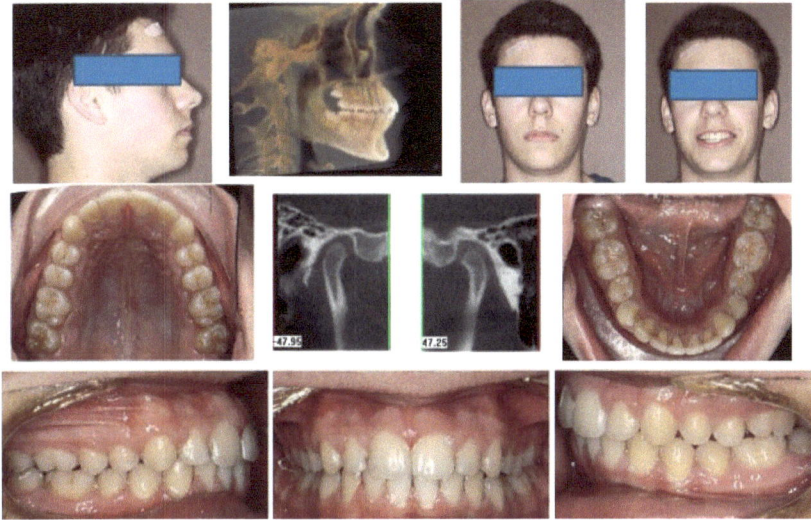

Fig. (7.14). Final records after 15 months treatment. It can be seen that profile has been improved compared to the patients' initial profile, buccal occlusion is class I, normal overbite and overjet. It can also be seen that tomograms confirmed that the patient is not posturing forward or having dual bite.

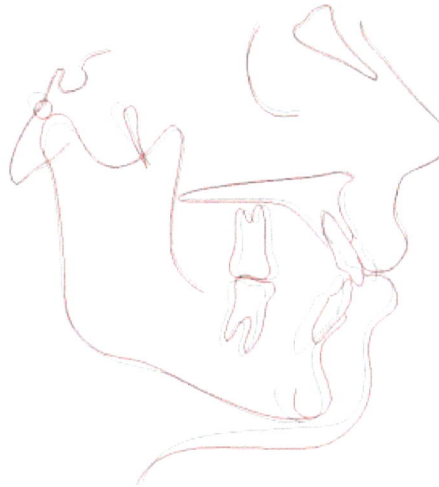

Fig. (7.15). Before and after treatment cephalometric analyses and superimposition reveal mandibular forward growth, improvement of apical base relationship due to improved mandibular forward projection/growth. Also maintenance of lower incisors angulation to mandibular plan could be a combination of slight proclination and labial root torque of lower incisors.

Table 7.3. Confirms improvement of the patient's skeletal class II relationship.

Variable	Before	After
NPogFH	93°	94°
FH to S-N	19°	19°
SNA	79°	77°
SNB	72°	73°
ANB	7°	4°
WITS	8mm	2mm
NAPog	11°	5°
FH to Me-Go	15°	16°
S-N to Me-Go	34°	35°
S-N to Occ.	16°	20°
N-S-Gn	67°	67°
1u to SN	115°	102°
Max1-NA	35.9°	24.6°
1u-NA	4mm	4mm
II	109.4°	123.2°
1l to Go-Me	103°	103°
Mand1-NB	27.5°	28.1°
1l-NB	6mm	7mm
1l to A-Pog	1mm	4mm
1l to A-Pog Ang.	24°	27°
Pog-NB	3mm	3mm
Nasolabial Angle	117°	115°

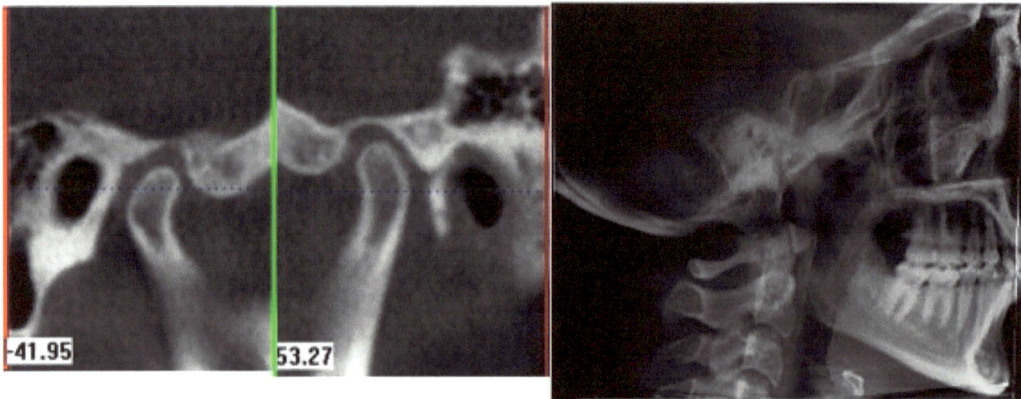

Fig. (7.16). Tomograms for another patient without wearing aligners. It can be seen that the anterior teeth were cut during this CBCT acquisition.

Another incident confirmed this effect. This incident had occured when a patient had a CBCT as part of the original records for Invisalign treatment (Fig. **7.16**), however the frontal part of the anterior teeth were cut during the CBCT scanning. To minimize exposure to radiation, a second set of x-ray was postponed until the appointment of Invisalign delivery. During the second set, the patient forgot to remove clear aligners during CBCT scanning (Fig. **7.17**). When comparing TMJ tomograms with and without clear aligners (Fig. **7.17**), it is obvious that the condyles when the patient wore clear aligners moved downward and forward as if the patient had had a functional appliance [5]. This could be just an assumption that clear aligners could be working as a full time function appliance assuming that the patients wear clear aligners all the time.

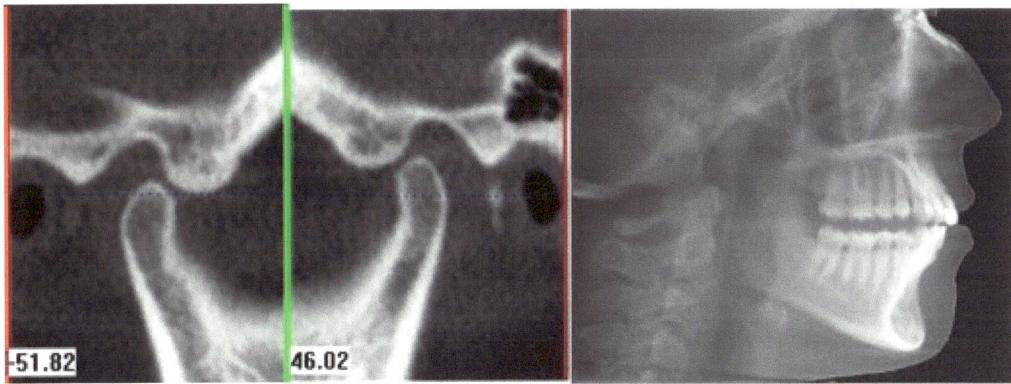

Fig. (7.17). Tomograms with patient wearing aligners. It can be seen that wearing clear aligners led to downward and forward positioning of the mandible simulating functional appliance wearing effect.

Case 3: Class II

This twelve-year-old female presented with skeletal class II due to retrognathic mandible and convex profile. Her chief complaint was to correct her overbite and overjet. Clinical records included CBCT-generated cephalometric radiographs confirmed skeletal class II relationship and class II division 1 malocclusion (full step class II buccal occlusion), 80% overbite and 6 mm overjet (Fig. **7.18**). Also, digital models showed upper 4 mm and lower 5 mm spacing (Fig. **7.19**).

Cephalometric analysis Table **7.4** showed initial class II as confirmed by increased ANB and increased Wits appraisal due to slightly prognathic maxilla and normally positioned mandible. Patient also showed forward growing mandible (Y-Axis) and low angle. Upper and lower incisors are slightly proclined as indicated from U1 - NA (°); L1 - NB (°) and IMPA (L1-MP) (°).

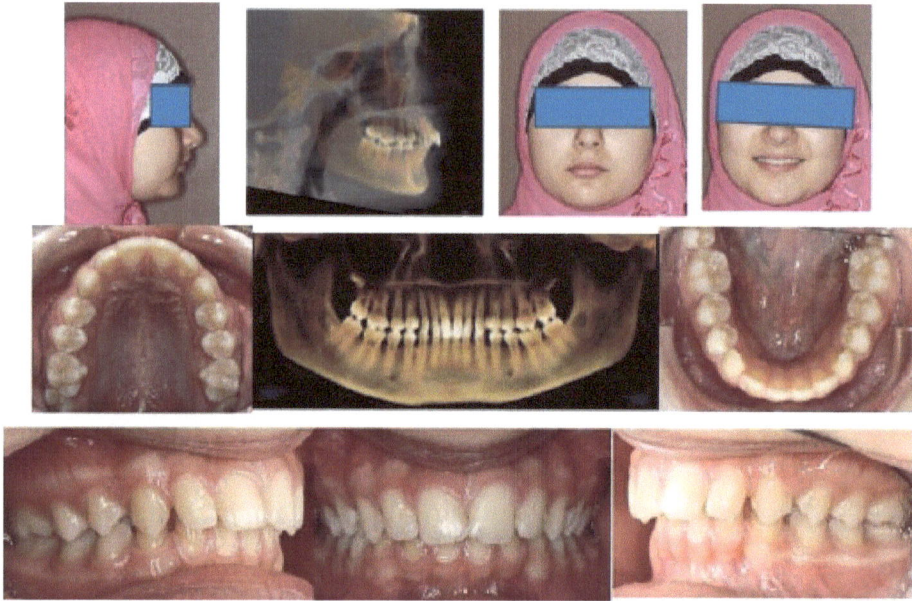

Fig. (7.18). A twelve-year old female with convex profile due to recessive chin with class II division 1 malocclusion. Overbite 80%, overjet 6 mm and spacing upper and lower dental arches.

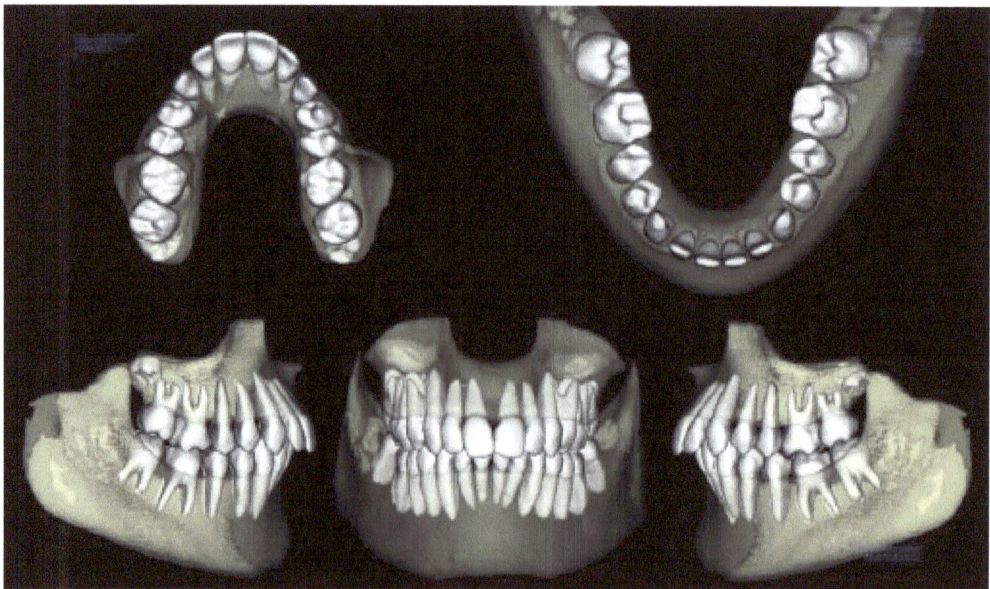

Fig. (7.19). CBCT-generated digital models using Anatomage software showing full step buccal occlusion, increased overjet and overbite with spaced upper and lower dental arches.

Table 7.4. Case II Class II before and after treatment.

		Initial	Final
Skeletal	SNA (°)	84.8	80
	SNB (°)	75.8	78.2
	ANB (°)	9	1.8
	Wits Appraisal (mm)	4.8	1.5
	Y-Axis -- Downs (SGn-FH) (°)	50	54
	FMA (MP-FH) (°)	14.5	18.3
	LFH/TFH (ANS-Me:N-Me) (%)	48.7	49.7
Dental	Interincisal Angle (U1-L1) (°)	115.8	146.7
	U1 - NA (mm)	2.5	-1.1
	U-Incisor Protrusion (U1-APo) (mm)	6.9	1.1
	U1 - NA (°)	28.2	9.9
	U1 - SN (°)	113	89.9
	L1 - NB (mm)	4.3	0.8
	L1 - NB (°)	29.4	19.1
	L1 - Occ Plane (°)	64.3	73
	IMPA (L1-MP) (°)	98.2	88.5
Soft Tissue	Lower Lip to E-Plane (mm)	-4.8	-3.6
	Upper Lip to E-Plane (mm)	-5.4	-3.3
	Nasolabial Angle (Col-Sn-UL) (°)	114.3	115.6

Treatment Planning

Patient had treatment planned by another orthodontist to have upper two premolar extraction and a headgear and full orthodontic treatment for two years by another orthodontist. Patient was given the options of full fixed orthodontic treatment or Invisalign treatment. The patient and her parents chose Invisalign treatment. Because of the recessive chin and the forward growth potential of the mandible, the treatment plan was to maximize forward growth potential by closing lower spaces by retracting lower incisors to allow for more overjet so that the mandible can grow forward. At the same time, to trigger mandibular growth, treatment planning involved slight distalization of upper molars utilizing class II elastics between upper canine cuts and buttons bonded to the buccal surface of the lower first molars. Patient was fitted with 46 aligners and was instructed to wear aligners 22 hours per day seven days a week and to change aligners every week if the patient felt that the aligners are loose.

Treatment Progress

At stage/aligner number 13 out of 46 aligners, clincheck showed edge-to-edge molar relationships on both sides. However, clinical photographs showed full step class I molar relationship on both sides. Also, profile showed improvement with chin projection improved forward compared to the initial records (Fig. **7.20**)

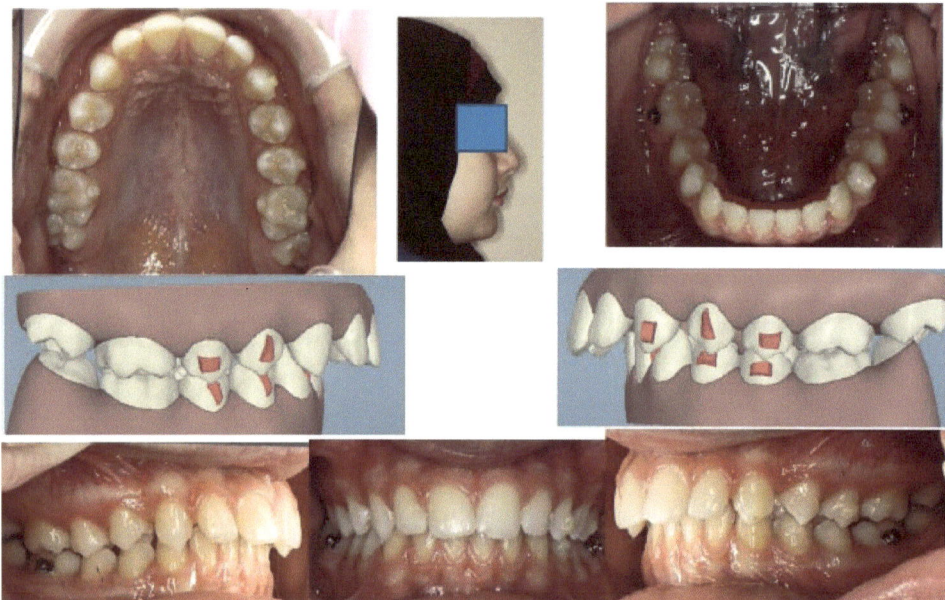

Fig. (7.20). Progress records showing improved molar relationships compared to proposed stage 13 clincheck. Also, patient's chin projection has been improved compared to initial profile photos.

At stage 46 aligners, it the patient's occlusion showed class I molars and canines, with slight deep bite (Fig. **7.21**, **7.22**). Also, patient's profile was improved to straight profile, and patient's head posture was improved giving even more forward chin projection than the initial or progress ones (Fig. **7.23**). Patient and parent did not prefer to continue improving overbite with refinement aligners.

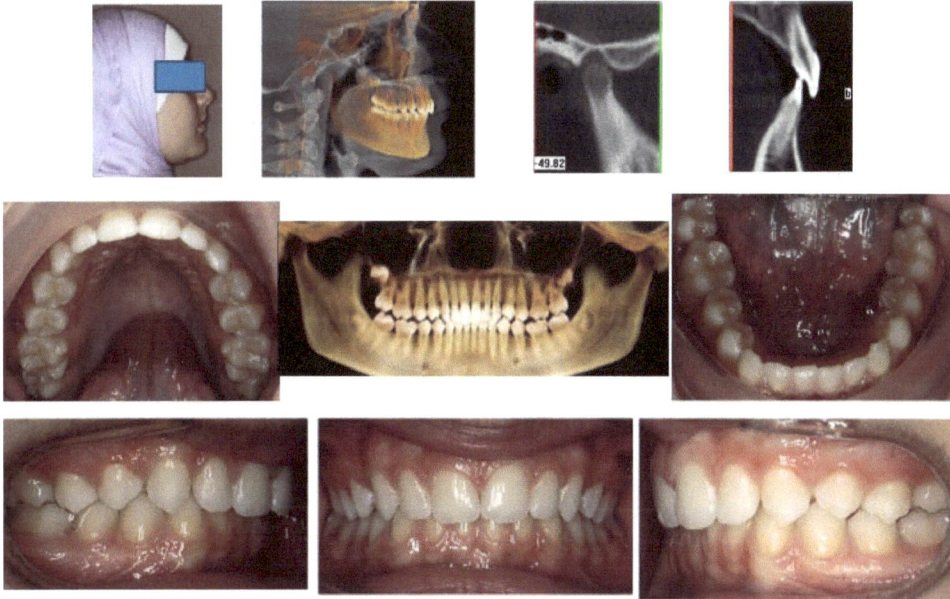

Fig. (7.21). Patient's final records showing improved profile, class I molars and canine relationships. Also, tomogram show that the patient was not posturing forward. CBCT-generated sagittal screens of upper and lower incisors showed that upper and lower incisors are situated normally within the alveolar bone.

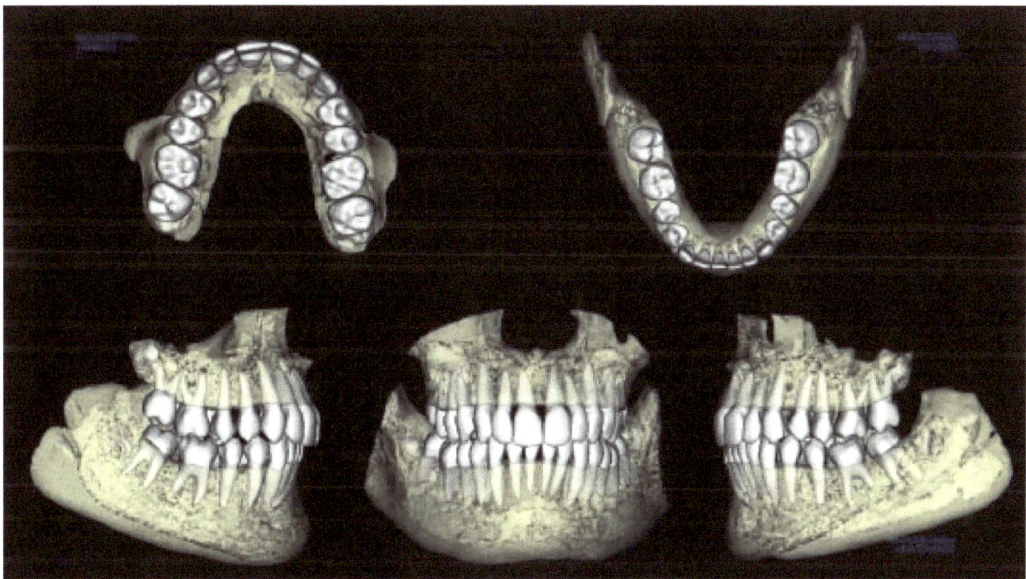

Fig. (7.22). Final CBCT-generated digital models.

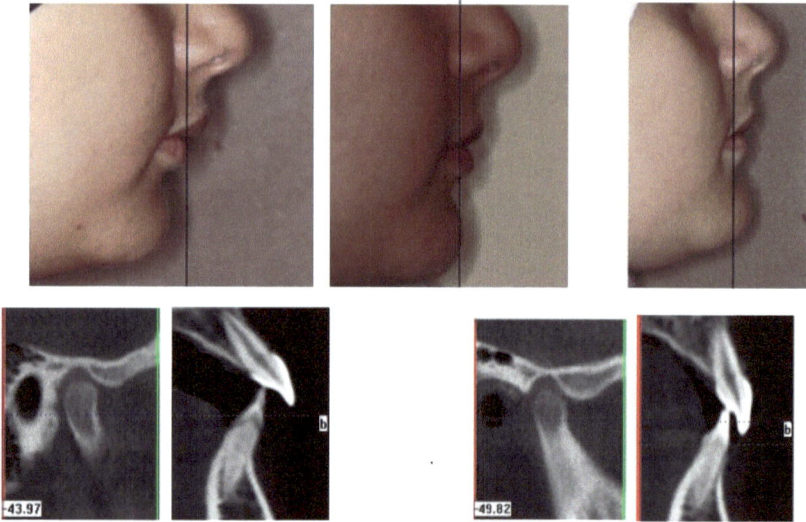

Fig. (7.23). Top row showing profile changes throughout the course of treatment as well as before and after tomograms and CBCT-generated sagittal screens of anterior teeth. It can be seen that there is major improvement of the patient's profile, especially chin projection between the initial and progress. At the end of the treatment, the patient's head posture has been improved which also gives more improvement of chin forward projection. It can also be seen that mandibular condyles after treatment are still in centric relationship within the condylar fossa (no forward shift or Sunday bite was observed) while axial inclination of the upper and lower front teeth are improved by Invisalign alone over 12 months of treatment.

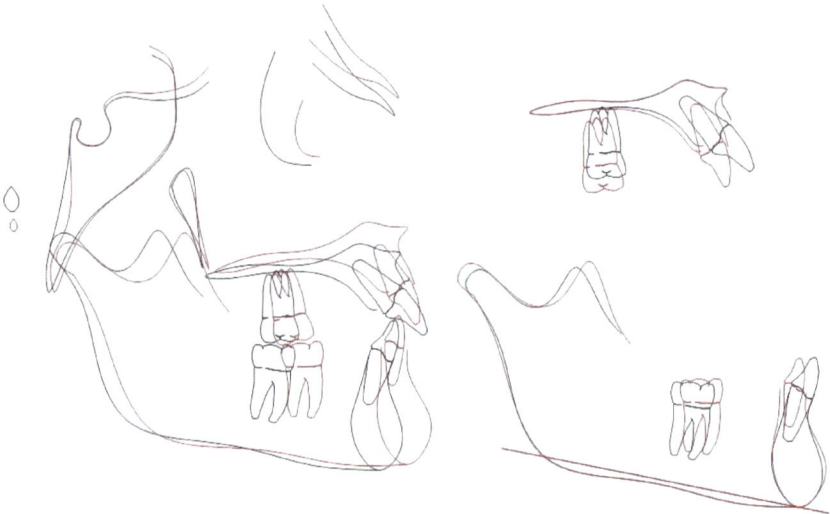

Fig. (7.24). Superimposition of before (black) and after (red) lateral cephalometric radiographs. The improvement in skeletal relationship is mainly due to mandibular forward growth. The overcorrection of incisors inclination was achieved by mandibular forward growth. This superimposition is in agreement with Bioprogressive technique (6).

Also, post treatment CBCT-driven sagittal screens of the upper and lower incisors show that lower incisors' crowns have been torqued lingually or roots torqued labially compared to original CBCT-driven sagittal screens of the same incisors. This could be retraction of upper incisors the end of treatment while the overbite was slightly deep. A critical review of this case, lower incisors should have been intruded at the same time they were retracted.

Post-treatment cephalometric analysis, Table **7.4** and Fig. (**7.24**) (Cephalometric superimposition) show improved skeletal relationship (ANB and Wits) and correction of upper and lower incisor inclinations.

Case 4: Class II

A 13 year-old boy was presented to our clinic with a chief complaint that he had a deep overbite and crooked teeth that needed to be fixed. Clinical records show straight profile with strong chin (Fig. **7.25**). Intraoral photos and clincheck show a full step class II molars/canines with 100% (Impinging) overbite. Patient had a 5 mm crowding in the upper arch and 2 mm crowding lower dental arch.

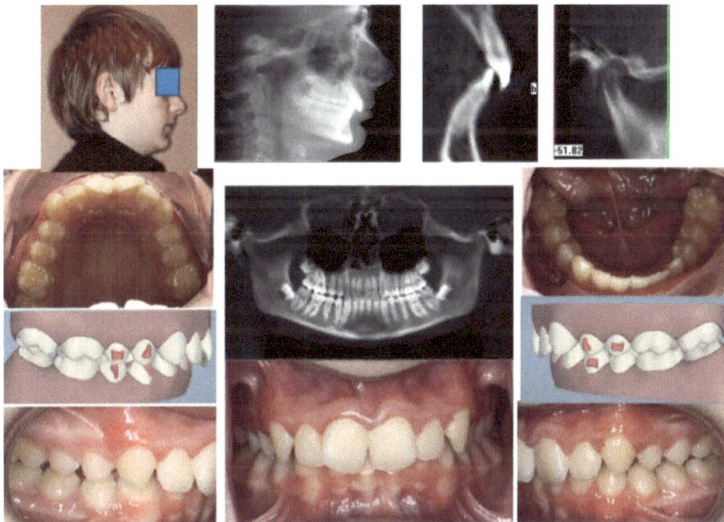

Fig. (7.25). Initial clinical records showing deep overbite, moderately crowded upper arch and minimum crowding in the lower arch. Although intraoral side photographs show end to end class II relationship, clincheck presents full step class II relationships of the canine and molars on the left side and class II end to end right molar and canine relationships.

Cephalometric analysis revealed class II tendency (Table **7.5**), Inter-incisal angle confirmed the clinical deep overbite.

Table 7.5. Before and after treatment cephalometric analyses of case 4, Class II deep overbite.

		Initial	Final
Skeletal	SNA (°)	83.2	78.4
	SNB (°)	78.7	77.3
	ANB (°)	4.5	1.1
	Wits Appraisal (mm)	3.6	-0.2
	Y-Axis -- Downs (SGn-FH) (°)	56.5	49.2
	FMA (MP-FH) (°)	18	8.9
	LFH/TFH (ANS-Me:N-Me) (%)	52.3	52.5
Dental	Interincisal Angle (U1-L1) (°)	139.8	126.6
	U1 - NA (mm)	2.1	3
	U-Incisor Protrusion (U1-APo) (mm)	3.1	2.2
	U1 - NA (°)	17.3	30.5
	U1 - SN (°)	100.5	108.9
	L1 - NB (mm)	1.2	1.3
	L1 - NB (°)	18.5	21.9
	L1 - Occ Plane (°)	71.5	71.3
	IMPA (L1-MP) (°)	97.3	100.9
Soft Tissue	Lower Lip to E-Plane (mm)	-3.4	-3.5
	Upper Lip to E-Plane (mm)	-5.6	-4
	Nasolabial Angle (Col-Sn-UL) (°)	165.5	115

Patient and parent were provided with two treatment option, 1) full fixed orthodontic treatment or 2) Invisalign treatment. Patient and parents were informed with advantages and disadvantages of each treatment modality.

Patient and parent chose Invisalign option. Treatment objectives were to improve facial profile if possible, improve class II malocclusion, specifically posterior occlusion and deep overbite as well as upper and lower crowding and axial inclination of the anterior teeth.

Patient was fitted with 48 aligners coupled with class II elastics. Half cusp molar distalization was prescribed, taking into consideration the mandibular distal shift that was seen in the initial tomograms (Fig. **7.26**). Patient was informed to wear aligners 20-22 hours/day and change them when they start to be loose, which normally happens after 1 week of full time wear.

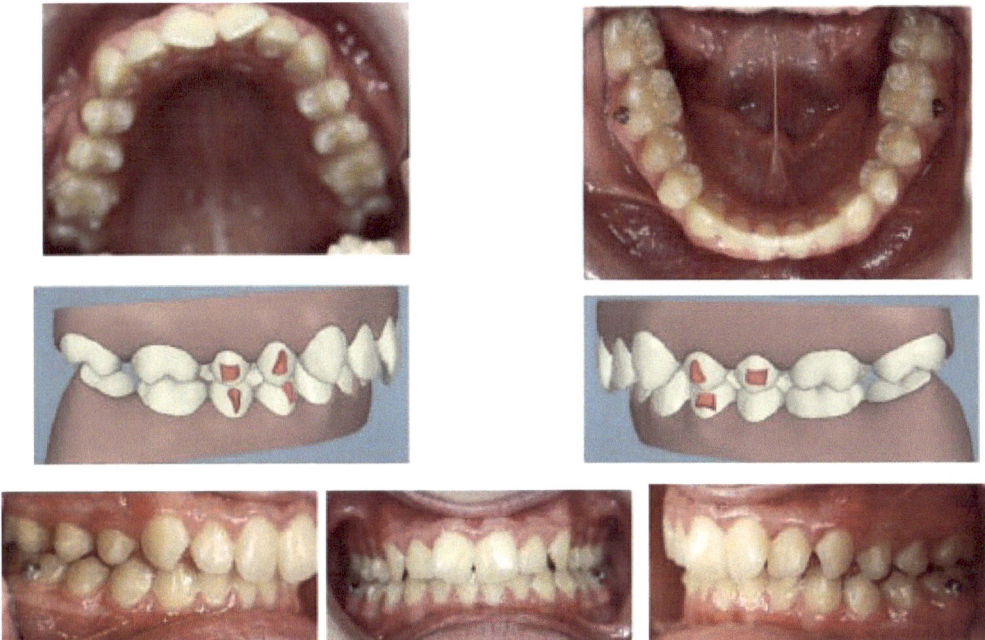

Fig. (7.26). Progress photos at stage 13/48. It can be seen that overbite as well as buccal occlusion have been improved compared to initial ones in figure 7.25.

Treatment Progress

At stage 13 out of 48 trays (four months and one week), the patient presented clinically with super class I molar relationship while clincheck shows stage 13 at end to end relationships. This could be due to the fact that clear aligners disengage the occlusion allowing the mandible to be projected forward into central relationship. In addition, deep overbite has been improved at this stage compared to the corresponding clincheck (Fig. **7.26**). At stage 48, patient was finished without refinement and intraoral photographs show full step class I molars and canine relationship, improved overbite and relieved upper and lower dental crowding (Fig. **7.27**).

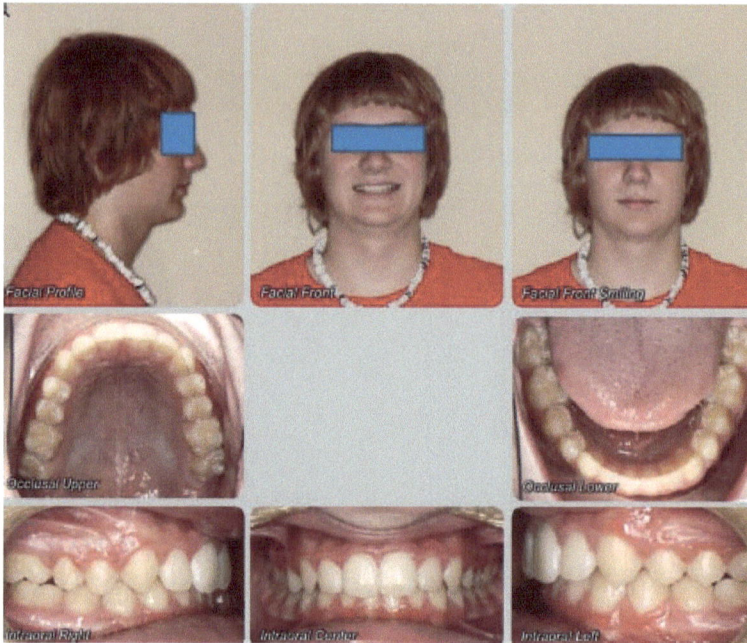

Fig. (7.27). Final clinical photographs showing class I molars and canines as well as improved overbite.

CRITICAL EVALUATION OF THE CASE

Although this case showing improvement in addressing the patient's initial chief concerns and finishing in a relatively short time, this case could have been managed better in terms of correcting class II without the need for upper molar distalization since initial distal shift was confirmed in the initial tomograms. Without upper molar distalization, we could have finished the case with more improved overbite compared to the achieved results and more forward projection of the chin. The distalization of the upper molars and consequently upper incisors distalization torqued lower incisors as can be seen from the CBCT-driven sagittal screens in (Figs. **7.28** and **7.29**). In such cases, class II correction might have been better started without upper molar distalization and informing the patient that refinement might be needed if we need more improvement of class II buccal occlusion than finishing with slightly retrognathic face.

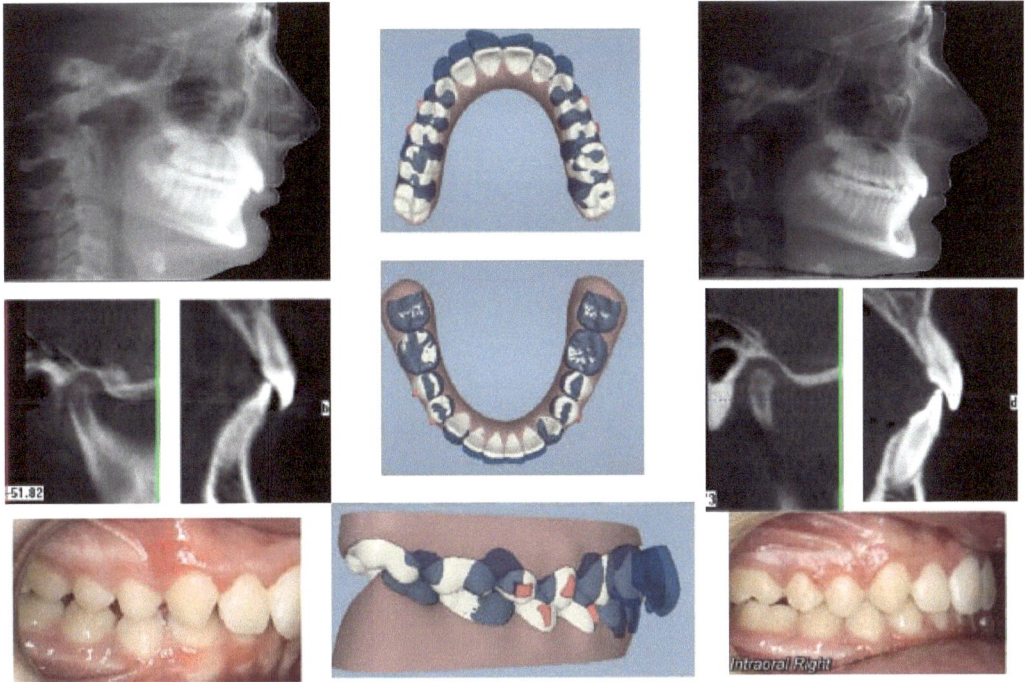

Fig. (7.28). Clincheck superimposition showing upper molar distalization and upper incisor retraction and intrusion. This confirms the changes from before (left column) to after treatment (right column).

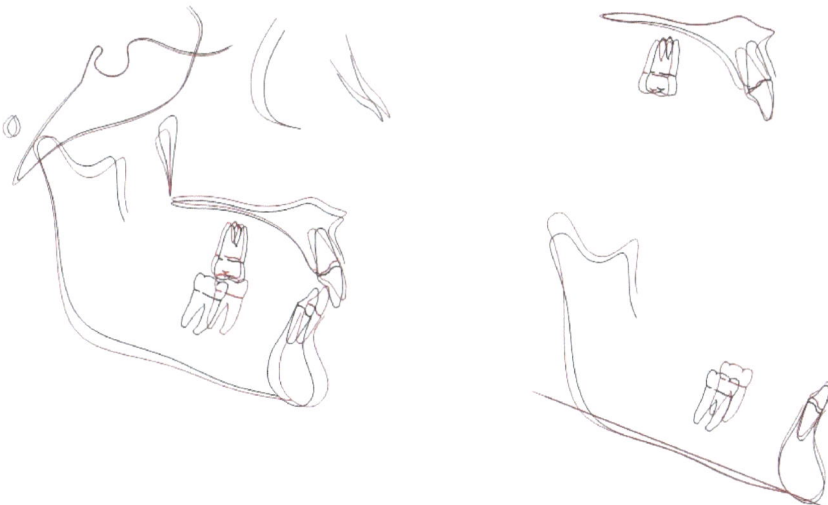

Fig. (7.29). Superimposition of before and after treatment cephalometric tracings of Case 4 Class II deep overbite.

In summary, CBCT seems to be crucial in diagnosis and treatment planning of class II cases, specifically in terms of detecting if there is any distal mandibular shift or not as well as providing real information about anterior alveolar bone width and how this can be used in determining type of tooth movement to be achieved.

In order to maintain or provide torque to upper incisors, counter movement may be needed before, during or after retracting upper incisors. Power ridges alone may not be enough in producing the effective required labial crown torque in deep overbite cases with severely retroclined upper incisors. As alternative, the clinician should order labial crown torque even before upper incisors lingual movement. This is of particular importance in cases where patients are initially presented with underdeveloped mandibles, in these cases labial crown torque provides an overjet for mandibular forward projection whether by allowing for forward mandibular growth in growing children or allowing appropriate axial inclination in adults prior to retracting upper incisors while maintaining a normal axial inclination (torque).

Upper molar distalization in teenagers or growing children can trigger faster forward mandibular projection, either can be interpreted as the forward arcial mandibular growth as Ricketts explained many years ago [6] when he used cervical head gear to extrude and distalize upper molars and consequently the occlusion is disengaged and the extruded upper molars can act as fulcrums to stimulate arcial forward mandibular growth. Upper molar distalization can also be interpreted as a fast track correction of molar and buccal occlusion than using class II elastics alone with forward bite jump.

Clear aligners also might be used as functional appliances. Our accidental discovery with two CBCT –generated tomograms scans with and without clear aligners wear proves that a functional appliance-like action can be produced by clear aligners.

REFERENCES

[1]   Boyd RL. Complex Orthodontic Treatment Using a New Protocol for the Invisalign Appliance. J Clin.
       Oorthod 2007; 9(XLI): 525-47.

[2]   Dahr S. Dr. Sam Daher's Techniques for Class II Correction with Invisalign and Elastics. Clinical tips and techniques by Align technology. 2011.

[3]   Schwartz A. Class II Deep Bite Correction with Invisalign CASE STUDY by Align Technology. 2010. M20139

[4]   Björk A. Prediction of mandibular growth rotation. Am J Orthod 1969; 55(6): 585-99.
[http://dx.doi.org/10.1016/0002-9416(69)90036-0] [PMID: 5253957]

[5]   Kinzinger G, Kober C, Diedrich P. Topography and morphology of the mandibular condyle during fixed functional orthopedic treatment --a magnetic resonance imaging study. J Orofac Orthop 2007; 68(2): 124-47.
[http://dx.doi.org/10.1007/s00056-007-0650-0] [PMID: 17372710]

[6]   Ricketts RM. Institute of Bioprogressive. Orthodontic treatment in the growing patient. Mechanics. 146-8.

CHAPTER 8

Treatment of Class III Malocclusion Using Clear Aligners

Abstract: Treatment of class III cases with clear aligners maybe a challenge. This is unlike class II where upper molars can be distalized or even do a functional appliance effect. Class III on the other hand, is different. In many growing cases, upper jaw may be required to move forward or restraining lower jaw forward growth in growing children is required. In adult patients, class III management is even more challenging. If a case presented with class III malocclusion that does not have a skeletal component, it can be manageable with clear aligners, however if there is a class III skeletal relationship, orthognathic surgery might be required. Clear aligners still may be used, however careful diagnosis and treatment planning as well as thorough communication with the patients and especially discussion of the treatment expectations is very important before, during and towards finishing of treatment.

Keywords: Camouflage, Class III, Control, Cross-bite, Malocclusion, Mechanics, Occlusal plan, Surgical corrections, Treatment planning, Vertical dimension.

INTRODUCTION

Class III management may include one of the following strategies: 1) only orthodontic management of the dental class III malocclusion would be aimed at camouflage treatment or backward rotation of the mandible which might help improvement of anteroposterior (AP) correction. However backward rotation of the mandible, although can be advantageous in cases with brachy or meso facial types. Backward rotation of the mandible is usually not recommended in cases with high angle or dolichofacial type. 2) Growth modification in growing children might be aimed at maximizing maxillary growth and harnessing, if possible, mandibular growth and 3) Orthognathic surgical treatment, which may involve maxillary forward surgical repositioning or mandibular surgical backward

Tarek El-Bialy, Donna Galante & Sam Daher

setback. In many cases, mandibular surgical backward setback may not be recommended in cases with compromised airway or patients having sleep disorders.

Boyd was the first to publish surgical-orthodontic treatment of two skeletal class III patients with Invisalign and fixed appliances [1]. In his protocol, pre-surgical decompensation of upper and lower incisors, coordination of upper and lower arches are done by Invisalign then a pre-surgical partial bonding with fixed appliance is used for intermaxillary fixation, then post-surgical finishing is done by Invisalign.

The possible use of clear aligners in growing class III cases includes: 1) using clear aligners with cuts for elastics to be hooked to face mask should maxillary protraction is an objective for a patient with maxillary deficiency, 2) camouflage treatment in adults if skeletal imbalance may be acceptable. This may be achieved by intermaxillary class III elastics, or 3) use clear aligners for preparation before surgical intervention to correct the skeletal class III malrelationship.

Case Presentation

This is a 16 years and 6 months old male who presented to our clinic with chief complaint that his front teeth are crowded and he had anterior cross bite. His medical history was non-contributory however his oral hygiene was fair and needed improvement. His profile was slightly convex with a dolichofacial type and slight hypermentalis muscle activity (Fig. **8.1**). Intraoral photographs and digital models (Fig. **8.2**) revealed a class III malocclusion with anterior and posterior cross bites. Also, patient presented with fair oral hygiene that was instructed to improve and visit his dentist for continuous cleanings and checkups. Cephalometric analysis (Table **8.1**) revealed class III skeletal with high mandibular angle. Also, cephalometric analysis revealed slightly protruded and proclined upper incisors while lower incisors were within normal range relative to NB plane, however lower incisors inclination to mandibular plane was reteroclined. These axial inclinations confirm the patient has a class III skeletal relationship as per the apical base discrepancy (ANB, WITS analyses).

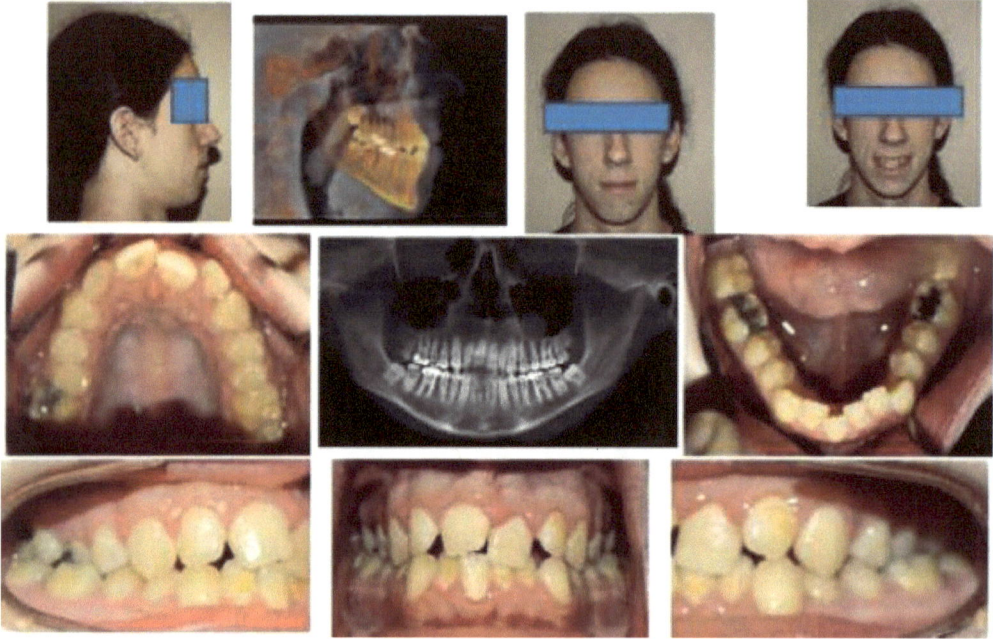

Fig. (8.1). Initial clinical photographs show dolichofacial type and hyper mentalis muscle activity. Also, intraoral photographs reveal class III malocclusion and fair oral hygiene.

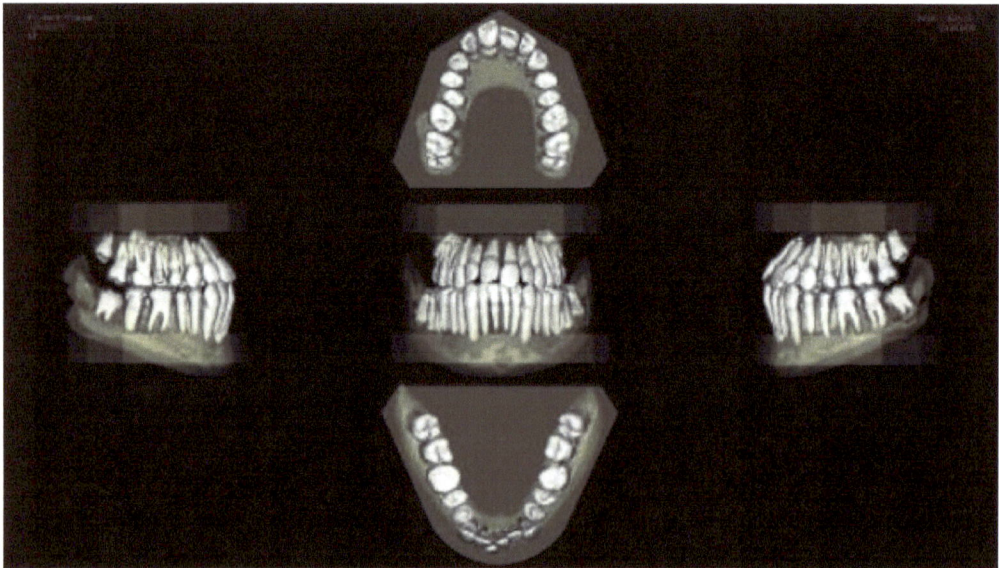

Fig. (8.2). Initial CBCT-generated digital models confirm class III malocclusion and anterior/posterior cross bite.

Table 8.1. Before and after treatment cephalometric analyses of class III case.

		Initial	Final
Skeletal	SNA (°)	81.9	80.9
	SNB (°)	80.8	79.1
	ANB (°)	1.1	1.8
	Wits Appraisal (mm)	-2.4	-0.2
	Y-Axis -- Downs (SGn-FH) (°)	59.8	60.7
	FMA (MP-FH) (°)	32.8	33.5
	LFH/TFH (ANS-Me:N-Me) (%)	58.5	57.9
Dental	Inter-incisal Angle (U1-L1) (°)	128.5	141.4
	U1 - NA (mm)	6.4	5.3
	U-Incisor Protrusion (U1-APo) (mm)	7.1	6.8
	U1 - NA (°)	29.3	24.8
	U1 - SN (°)	111.2	105.8
	L1 - NB (mm)	5.9	2.5
	L1 - NB (°)	21.1	11.9
	L1 - Occ Plane (°)	73.3	80.7
	IMPA (L1-MP) (°)	79.7	67.8
Soft Tissue	Lower Lip to E-Plane (mm)	0.1	-3.2
	Upper Lip to E-Plane (mm)	-5.2	-8.3
	Nasolabial Angle (Col-Sn-UL) (°)	112	121.7

Digital models confirm the presence of full step class III malocclusion and the patient has an increased mandibular total Bolton discrepancy of 3 mm. Also, the patients presented with upper second premolars were in cross bite due to slightly constricted upper and wide lower dental arches. In addition, he had lower 4 mm crowding and upper 4 mm spacing.

Treatment objectives were to maintain his facial profile and skeletal relationships since the patient declined surgery and accepted compromised treatment. Also, other objectives were to improve his anterior and posterior cross bites, improve upper and lower crowding, and improve his class III occlusal relationships if possible.

Initial Treatment Plan

Initial treatment plan was to close upper spaces by expanding upper arch as well as moving upper buccal segments forward in order to correct class III buccal occlusion and to relieve lower crowding using interproximal reduction due to the existing Bolton discrepancy. Initial set of aligners included 15 aligners that should have provided improvement in upper and lower misaligned teeth close upper spaces, treat upper premolars cross bite and improve upper buccal class III occlusion.

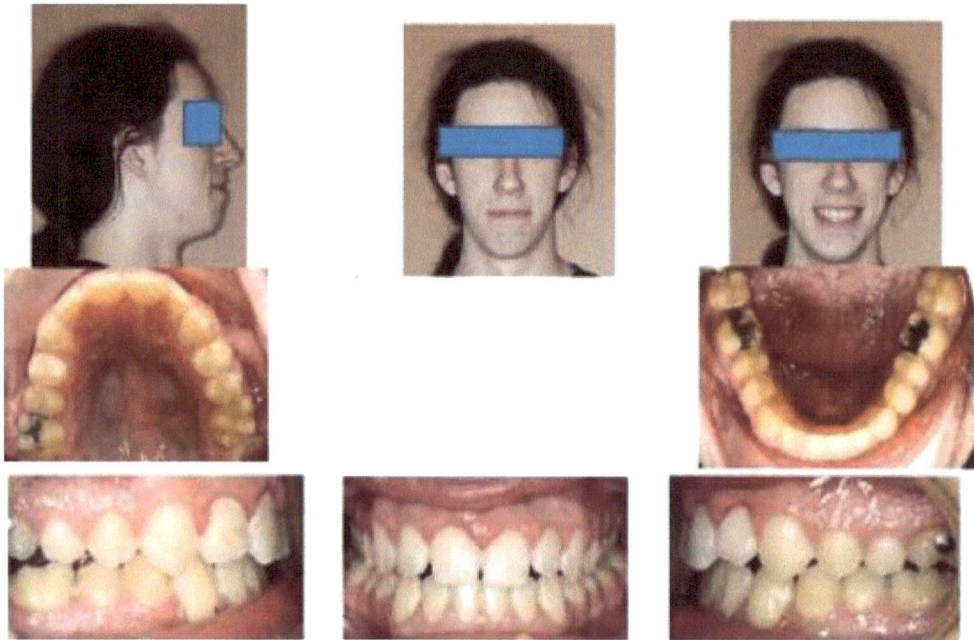

Fig. (8.3). Class III case after treatment showing balanced face and full step class I posterior and canine relationships. Left side canine relationship shows over correction to an edge-to-edge class II (over correction).

Results: After this initial treatment phase, left canine relationship was class I, upper and lower teeth crowding, upper second premolars cross bites were improved but not fully corrected. Refinement (additional aligners) phase was then prescribed and accepted by the patient utilizing class III elastics and consisted of 17 aligners. The patient was compliant with elastic wearing and aligners as well.

At the end of the refinement, the patient showed class II end to end relationship on the left canine and full class I relationship of the right canine and improvement of both buccal segments into class I relationship (Fig. **8.3**).

Cephalometric analyses (Table **8.1**) and superimposition (Fig. **8.4**) of before and after treatment show maintenance of the ANB angle while Wits appraisal was improved. Class III was mainly improved by reteroclination of lower incisors, while upper incisors' position and inclination were improved. Although mandibular plane angle was slightly increased, this did not affect the whole face/profile. Cephalometric superimposition is in agreement with the cephalometric analyses in terms of reteroclination of lower incisors while posterior class III malocclusion was improved by forward movement of the upper posterior teeth as seen in the cephalometric superimposition (Fig. **8.4**),

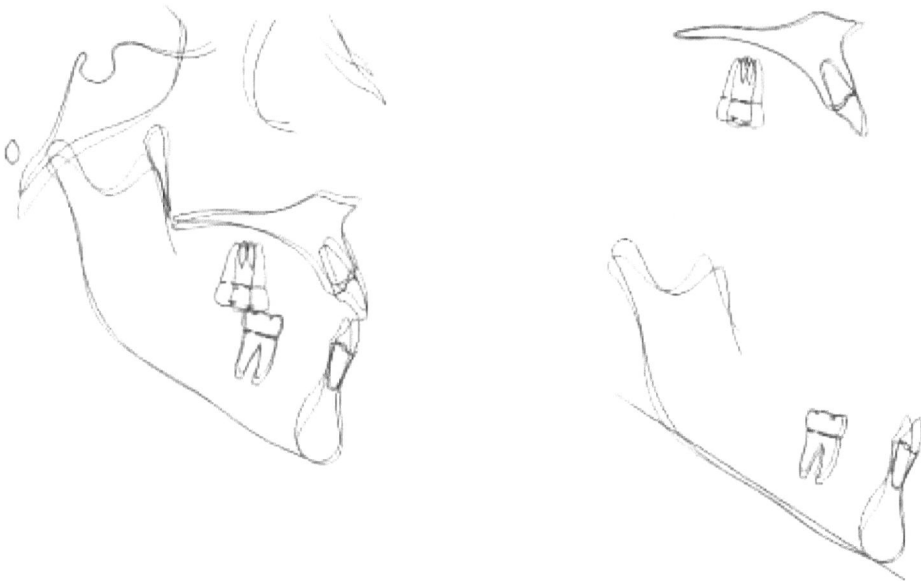

Fig. (8.4). Superimposition of before (black) and after (red) treatment cephalometric tracings. It can be seen that lower incisors were reteroclined correcting anterior relationship and upper molars moved forward correcting class III buccal occlusion.

DISCUSSION

In class III skeletal and dental malocclusion, camouflage treatment may be directed to more compensation of the teeth, however it has been shown that in class III skeletal relationship, camouflage treatment can lead to severe root resorption and/or compromised periodontal health [2, 3]. In order to provide better axial inclination, it has been recommended to add reverse torque to the upper incisors (labial root torque) to minimize possible side effects referred to in [2, 3]. This can be produced with fixed orthodontic appliance by using low torque brackets in the upper anterior teeth. While using clear aligners, labial root torque can be achieved by retroclination of upper incisors, normally this will lead to labial root torque, prescribe labial root torque or extrude upper incisors. All these techniques can produce labial root torque of the upper incisors. When using class III elastics, there is always tendency for upper incisors to tip forward, or in other words, palatal root torque. Requesting incisor lingual crown torque would counteract the palatal root torque due to class III elastics. This can be seen in the improvement of upper incisors inclination in table 4 (cephalometric analysis) as well as in Fig. (**8.3**) (Cephalometric superimposition).

Summary of Class III Biomechanics

While planning mechanics for class III malocclusion correction, labial root torque of upper incisors can be achieved by retroclination of the upper incisors' crowns. The reverse can be done in the lower incisors. However, in some cases, lingual controlled tipping of lower incisors can also help correcting anterior cross bite or edge-to-edge relationship.

Controlled tipping can be achieved by clear aligners by applying counter moment that is aimed at counter effect the moment due to force. This can be easily achieved by applying lingual root torque to the lower incisors.

REFERENCES

[1]   Boyd RL. Surgical-orthodontic treatment of two skeletal Class III patients with Invisalign and fixed appliances. J Clin Orthod 2005; 39(4): 245-58.
[PMID: 15888956]

[2]   Mulie RM, Hoeve AT. The limitations of tooth movement within the symphysis, studied with

laminagraphy and standardized occlusal films. J Clin Orthod 1976; 12(10): 882-93-6-9.

[3]   Ten Hoeve A, Mulie RM. The effect of antero-postero incisor repositioning on the palatal cortex as studied with laminagraphy. J Clin Orthod 1976; 10(11): 804-822, 886-889.
        [PMID: 1069732]

CHAPTER 9

Treatment of Anterior Open Bite Using Clear Aligner Therapy

Abstract: Anterior open bite can be of dental, skeletal, functional or a combination of all three in origin. An anterior open bite is present when there is no contact between the upper and lower anterior teeth and no overbite (vertical overlap of the upper and lower incisors). The severity of open bite varies from an edge to edge relationship to a severe open bite with teeth contact only in the molar areas. Ideally, treatment of open bites should be started as early as they are diagnosed by the dentist or pediatric dentist/orthodontist. Often, early intervention can eliminate the causes of the open bite especially if they are related to a persistent habit such as thumb sucking or mouth breathing. Also, early intervention can re-direct jaw growth and establish a more favorable mandibular growth direction. This chapter will discuss treatment of open bite in non-growing patients by using clear aligner therapy and no adjunct orthognathic surgery.

Keywords: Anterior open bite, Clear aligners, Control, Edge-to-edge bite, Habit, Intrusion/extrusion, Mouth breathing, Tongue thrusting, Vertical dimension.

INTRODUCTION

Digit sucking is a common cause of anterior open bite. The incidence of digit sucking is around 30% at age 1 and decreases to 2% by age 12 [1]. Open bites that exist in the primary dentition usually will resolve on their own once the child ceases the digit habit. Anterior open bites that extend into the mixed and permanent dentition may require orthodontic or even surgical intervention. A vertical component to growth may occur during this time frame as the child persists with a digit habit, lip or tongue habits, airway obstruction and genetic skeletal growth abnormalities. Complex orthodontic treatment involving the use of molar intrusion with or without temporary anchorage devices may be required.

Tarek El-Bialy, Donna Galante & Sam Daher

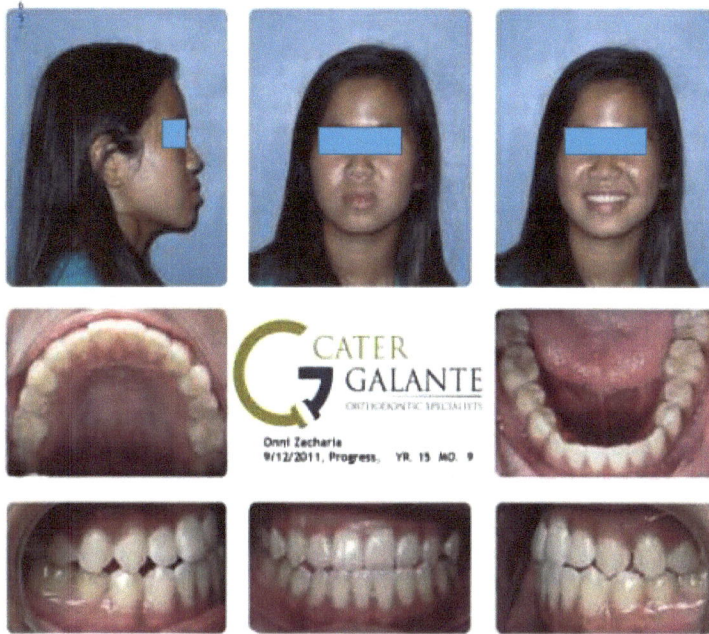

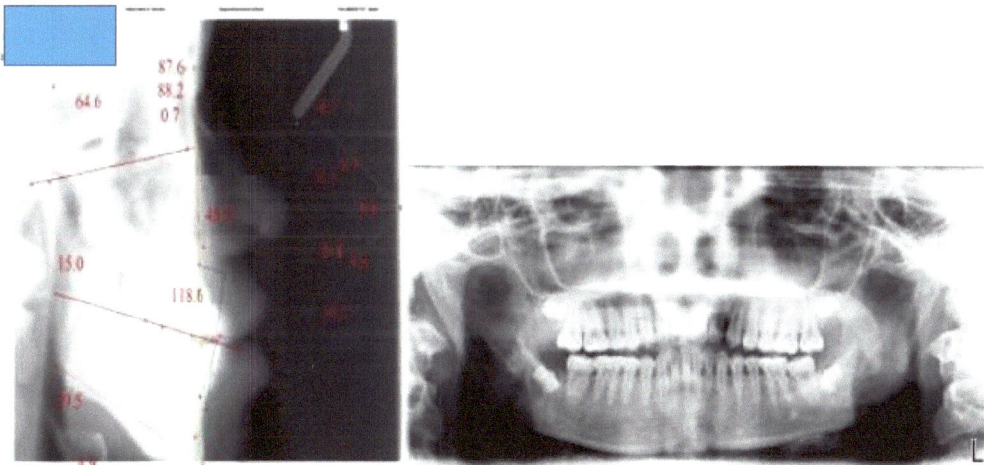

Fig. (9.1). Pretreatment clinical records A) photographs showing class III right side and anterior open bite/edge-to edge relationship. B) Initial Cephalometric and panoramic radiographs

Orthognathic surgery is often the last resort in treating these type of cases [2]. Fixed appliance therapy has been the standard of care in orthodontics in correcting anterior open bites. Unfortunately, research has shown that relapse is frequent with about 40 to 80% relapse [3 - 5]. Persistent anterior tongue position is often cited as one of the most important factors in relapse. Great success has been demonstrated by Dr. Robert Boyd, Chairman of the Department of Orthodontics at the University of Pacific Dental School, with use of clear aligners to treat anterior open bites [6]. This case study will show how clear aligners can predictability close anterior open bite.

CASE 1

A 16 year old female presented to our office with her mother with the chief compliant of a bite problem and not being able to chew properly. Medical history was non-contributory. Her dental history included a previous phase of treatment in the mixed dentition for "several years" while living in Asia. Mom stated that her bite was perfect at the end of that treatment and all her teeth were in place when the braces were removed. Since moving back to the United States, she has grown a few more inches and her bite changed. The patient was not interested in braces or treatment at all, but was more inclined to proceed with Invisalign than fixed appliances. Initial records (Fig. **9.1**) show that the patient has a mesiocephalic face (concave profile and prognathic chin projection) with a midline deviation to the left of approximately 3mm. She has an edge to edge anterior open bite and presents with a Class III molar relationship on the left side. Cephalometric analysis shows a significant class III skeletal pattern, high mandibular plane angle and bimaxillary protrusion of both upper and lower incisors.

Treatment Objectives

A non-extraction approach was presented to the patient and parent. Treatment objectives were to correct the edge-to edge open bite, reduce the bimaxillary protrusion, provide overjet and overbite and align the midlines.

Treatment Plan

Patient did not want to go through fixed orthodontic treatment again and was even reluctant to start Invisalign. However, her mother wanted her to have the bite problem corrected once and for all. She consented to wear clear aligners the required 22 hours a day along with any necessary elastics. Patient was given an initial set of 20 upper and lower aligners which were for worn 20 hours per day and changed every 2 weeks. Class III elastics were given to her at aligner 6 and worn on both sides. A refinement scan was performed with the iTero™ and a second set of 12 aligners was given to the patient along with a class III elastic on right side (Fig. **9.2**).

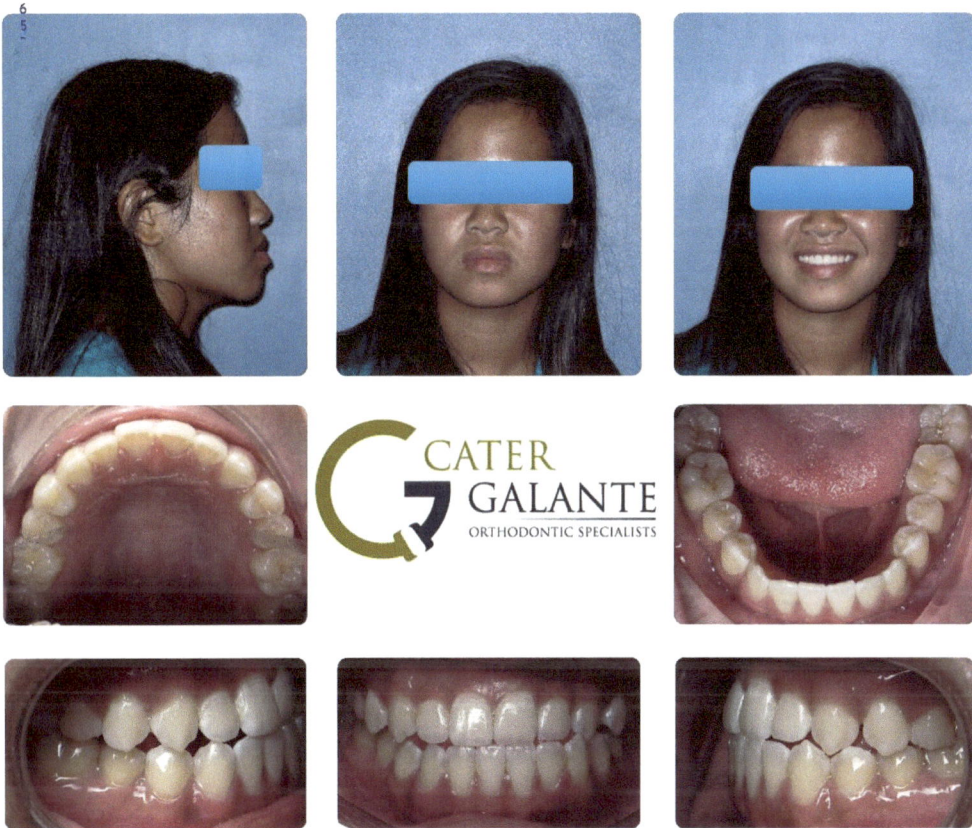

Fig. (9.2). Progress photos showing improvement of the right side Class III and buttons for class III elastics.

Total treatment time was 16 months. During the refinement stage, patient was instructed to change her aligners every 7 days. Final photos (Fig. **9.3**).

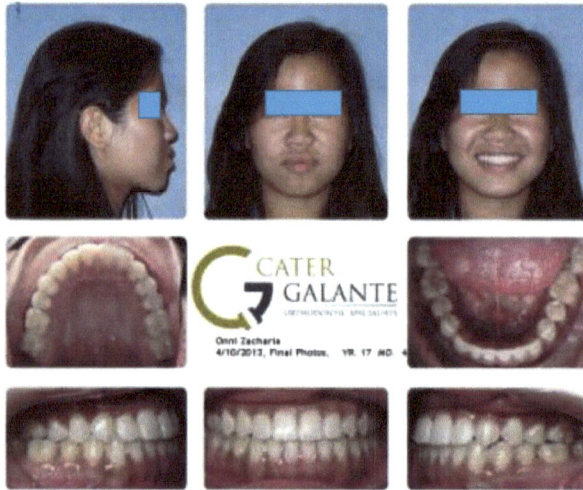

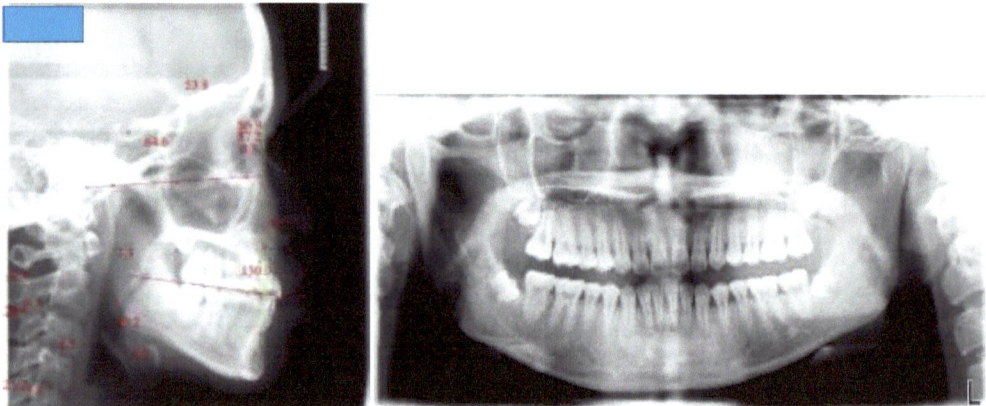

Fig. (9.3). A) Final Photos showing interdigitation of the right side into class I and improvement of anterior overbite and overjet. B) Final cephalometric and panoramic radiographs.

Patient was given an in house set of Essix retainers to wear 16 hours a day for 6 months, then 12 hours a day for the next 6 months. Retainer follow-up appointments in our office are scheduled every 3 to 4 months.

Discussion

The end result of 16 months of aligner wear resulted in approximately 2mm or overbite and 2mm of overjet along with alignment of the midlines and a solid class 1 molar and canine relationship. Pre and post panoramic views confirm the position of all permanent teeth including the positioning of the lower second molars which were tipped slightly mesially in the beginning of the treatment (Fig. **9.3**).

The cephalometric tracings and analyses show an improvement on the protrusion of the anterior teeth from an interincisal angle of 118.6 to 130.0. The SL line went from 48.9 degrees (slight clockwise rotation) to 53.8 degrees (slight counter-clockwise rotation) which indicated that the aligner therapy did not open the bite as would have occurred with traditional fixed appliances. Go-Gn/Sn did not change significantly either, further supporting the theory of intrusive force on the posterior teeth while the anterior teeth are being extruded [6].

Dr. Robert Boyd at the University of Pacific has published a comprehensive study of 32 successfully treated patients with anterior open bites and concluded that with clear aligner therapy bite force is increased on the posterior teeth due to aligner thickness in this area.

This accounts for posterior intrusion that is seen in many aligner open bite cases. Furthermore, he hypothesized that the tongue, which plays a major part in the relapse on anterior open bites, is permanently blocked out during treatment and may be moved distally due to the effect of the aligners on the lingual of the anterior teeth. The enhanced optimized attachments provided by Invisalign, are also helpful in extruding the anterior teeth predictably according to Dr. Boyd [6].

CASE 2

This is a 25-year old female who was referred by a neuromuscular dentist that stabilized her mandibular position in a downward and forward position to relieve her TMJ pain with an orthotic. After 8 months in treatment with the myofunc-tional orthotic, she was referred by her dentist to our office to close her open bite so that she would not need to wear the orthotic anymore in the future. In order to stabilize her lower jaw position obtained by the orthotic, a posterior build up was performed on the lower second molars that led to an anterior open bite extends from the right first molar to the left first molars (Fig. **9.4**). Initial photos, CBCT-driven lateral cephalometric, panoramic and tomograms confirmed that open bite with the mandibular condyles are in downward and forward position obtained by the myofunctional orthotic (Figs. **9.4** & **9.5**).

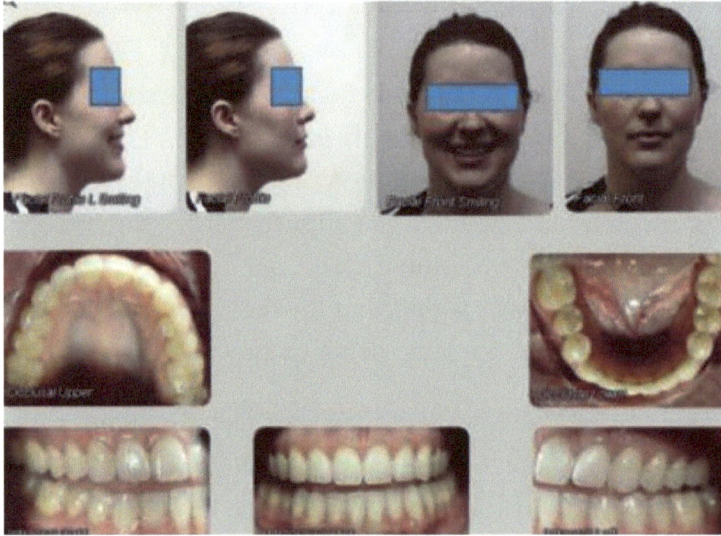

Fig. (9.4). Initial photos of case 2 showing anterior open bite that extends from the right first molars to the left first molars.

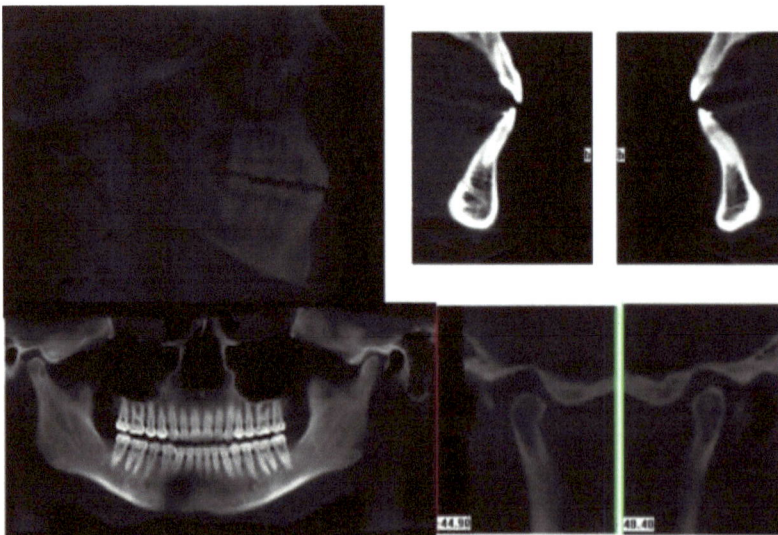

Fig. (9.5). Initial CBCT-driven lateral cephalometric, sagittal screens of the anterior teeth, panoramic and tomograms of case 2 showing anterior open bite that extends from the right first molars to the left first molars as well as the downward and forward position of the mandibular condyles within the TMJ fossa.

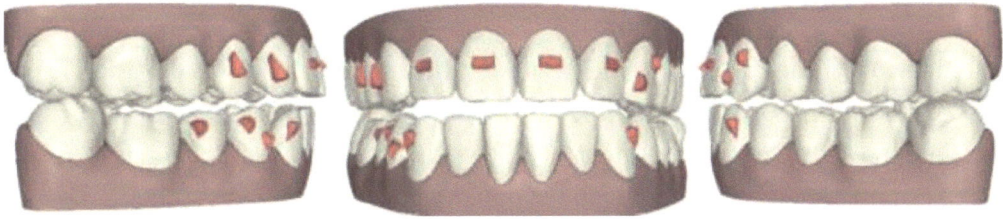

Fig. (9.6). Clincheck of case 2 showing the extrusion attachments applied to the anterior teeth and confirming the open bite that extends from the right first molars to the left first molars.

Treatment and Progress

Treatment included Invisalign treatment with extrusion attachments that were prescribed to the anterior teeth to extrude upper incisors and to close the open bite (Fig. **9.6**). The posterior teeth were allowed to spontaneous extrusion without attachments. The whole treatment comprises 23 aligners that the patient changed every week. After 7 months in treatment, the open bite was closed and the patient sought fine detailing of her occlusion (Fig. **9.7**).

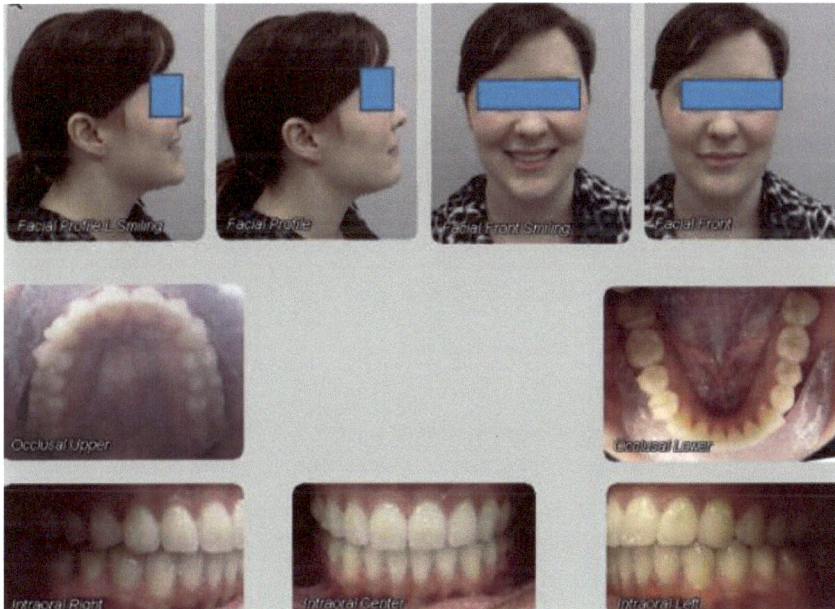

Fig. (9.7). Clinical photographs of case 2 after 7 months in treatment confirming closing the open bite.

Summary and Discussion

In summary, open bite cases can be treated with more predictability using clear aligners once the appropriate attachments and habit control management strategies are implemented. In particular, anterior teeth extrusion is always recommended, especially upper anterior teeth and posterior teeth can be intruded simultaneously. It is not recommended to extrude lower anteriors as this would lead to early aging faces. Vertical elastics can be prescribed on buttons attached to the canines as needed. Anterior tongue thrusting habit breaking appliance (like myofunctional mouth guards) is recommended to be used by patients 2-3 hours during the day to and during sleep train the tongue with the appropriate position. Other options to correct open bite include the use of temporary anchorage devices (TADs) buccal and palatal to the aligners while patients wear elastics between the buccal and palatal elastics TADs over the occlusal surfaces of the teeth.

REFERENCES

[1]   Burford D, Noar JH. The causes, diagnosis and treatment of anterior open bite. Dent Update 2003; 30(5): 235-41.
        [PMID: 12861760]

[2]   Ngan P, Fields HW. Open bite: a review of etiology and management. Pediatr Dent 1997; 19(2): 91-8.
        [PMID: 9106869]

[3]   Smithpeter J, Covell D Jr. Relapse of anterior open bites treated with orthodontic appliances with and without orofacial myofunctional therapy. Am J Orthod Dentofacial Orthop 2010; 137(5): 605-14.
        [http://dx.doi.org/10.1016/j.ajodo.2008.07.016] [PMID: 20451779]

[4]   Zuroff JP, Chen SH, Shapiro PA, Little RM, Joondeph DR, Huang GJ. Orthodontic treatment of anterior open-bite malocclusion: stability 10 years postretention. Am J Orthod Dentofacial Orthop 2010; 137(3): 302.e1-8.
        [PMID: 20197159]

[5]   Remmers D, Van't Hullenaar RW, Bronkhorst EM, Bergé SJ, Katsaros C. Treatment results and long-term stability of anterior open bite malocclusion. Orthod Craniofac Res 2008; 11(1): 32-42.
        [http://dx.doi.org/10.1111/j.1601-6343.2008.00411.x] [PMID: 18199078]

[6]   Comparison of Invisalign with Conventional Orthodontic Treatment for Anterior Open Bite Malocclusion. Dr Robert Boyd, Chairman of the Department of Orthodontics, University of the Pacific. 2011.

CHAPTER 10

Treatment of Facial Asymmetry Using Clear Aligners

Abstract: There are many etiological factors that could be attributed to facial skeletal asymmetry, including but not limited to hemifacial microsomia, unilateral temporomandibular joint ankylosis especially in growing patients or hypertrophic condyle on one side due to local tumor. Functional facial asymmetry could be attributed to bilateral constricted maxilla and the patient shifts his/her mandible to one side to achieve a comfortable occlusion on one side, or it could be due to dental interference, which mainly occurs due to one tooth in cross bite, usually upper lateral incisor. In this case, treatment is recommended as soon as possible especially in growing subjects to eliminate dental interference or to expand the maxilla so that no possible remodeling can happen in both TMJ fossae and possible need for surgical intervention later in life to fix jaw asymmetry. This chapter will discuss in details careful diagnosis of a case with facial asymmetry to simplify treatment planning.

Keywords: CBCT, Chin deviation, Crossbite, Elastics, Facial symmetry, Functional shift, Root movement, Stability, Tipping, Tomogrms.

INTRODUCTION

Lateral mandibular functional shift in the mixed dentition has been recommended to be treated as early as possible to eliminate possible permanent changes in the TMJ and fossa [1 - 9]. It has been reported that in growing children with lateral functional shift due to bilateral maxillary constriction or due to dental interference, treatment of unilateral cross bite can lead to self-correction of the lateral shift and this treatment and correction of condylar position in the glenoid fossa that may minimizing the need for orthognathic surgical correction in the future [4, 7, 8]. Tomograms confirm abnormal condylar position in both sides in cases with functional mandibular shift [4, 7, 8]. Another study showed that

Tarek El-Bialy, Donna Galante & Sam Daher

unilateral posterior crossbite can lead to asymmetric mandibular ramus height [6]. This study however is questionable as they used panoramic radiograph in assessing ramal height. Panoramic radiographs are known to have measurement errors due to the inherited magnification errors. Tomograms seem to be the best method of confirming mandibular condylar position before and after treatment.

Treatment of unilateral posterior crossbite may be performed using palatal expansion appliances (either removable or fixed), full fixed appliances with coordinated upper and lower archwires and/or crossbite elastics [10]. This chapter will show that functional mandibular shift once diagnosed and confirmed, can be treated as simple as removable appliance may be used to treat similar cases.

CASE PRESENTATION

This is a 39 years old female who presented to our clinic with a chief complaint that her dentist is referring her for comprehensive orthodontic treatment and surgical correction of her facial asymmetry. History revealed that the patient had no medical concern and she was initially interested in Invisalign treatment as fixed orthodontic braces were too challenging for her. However, her dentist who is an Invisalign provider convinced her that she is not a candidate for Invisalign treatment due to the high likelihood of surgical intervention and she better have comprehensive orthodontic treatment by an orthodontist and jaw surgery by an oral and maxillofacial surgeon. Clinical records (Fig. **10.1**) revealed that the patient had a balanced face with chin deviated to the patient's right side. Intraoral photographs show that the patient has cross bite of upper right lateral incisor and right buccal segment. Usually, cases with unilateral posterior cross bites develop facial asymmetry especially when the unilateral cross bite leads to lateral mandibular shift. In growing children, it is believed that fixing unilateral cross bite would lead to self-correction of the lateral shift and the possibility of minimizing the potential for the need of surgical intervention when the patient grows up beyond adulthood.

To confirm if the patient had skeletal asymmetry or functional shift, tomograms would be required. The advantage of CBCT is that tomograms are simply generated. Evaluation of the patient's initial CBCT generated tomograms

(Fig. **10.2**) confirmed the functional shift.

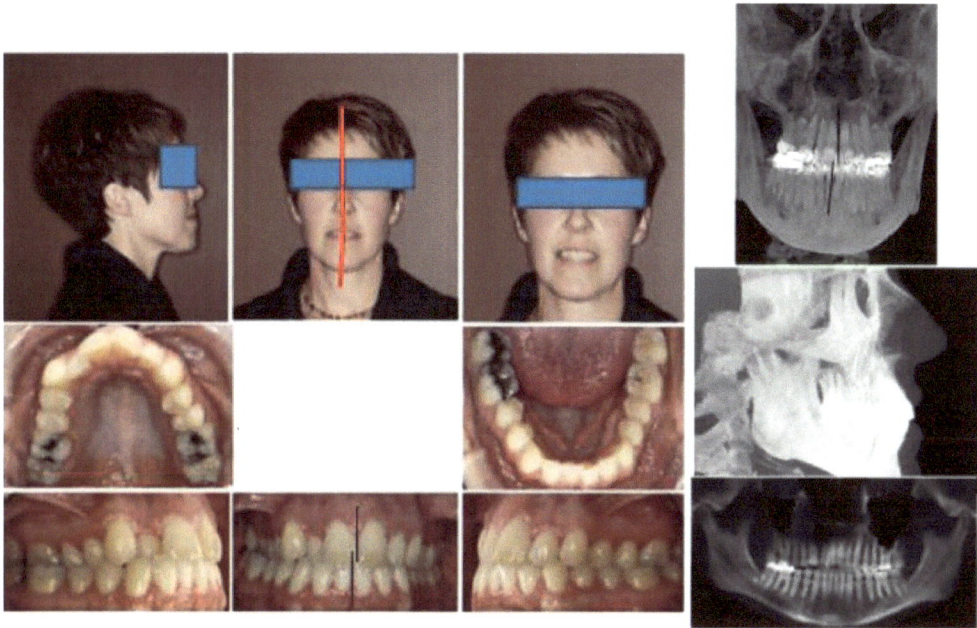

Fig. (10.1). Initial clinical records of the patient with facial asymmetry. CBCT generated frontal cephalometric radiograph showing shift of the chin to the patient's right side.

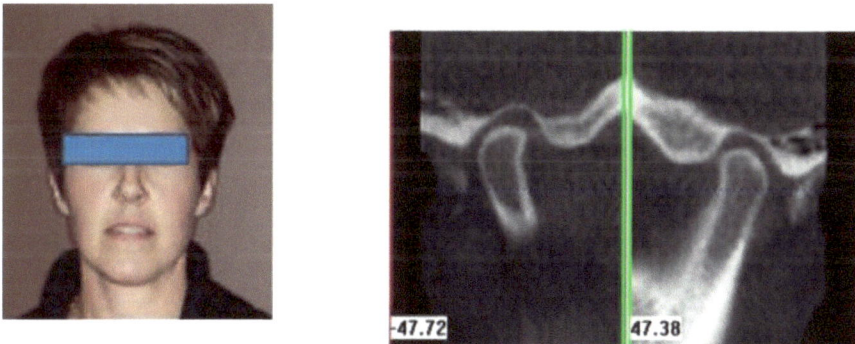

Fig. (10.2). Initial tomograms showing functional shift as the right side condyle of the patient has a posterior shift, while left condyle showing forward shift. The shifts are confirmed by comparing anterior and posterior disk spaces on each side.

Lateral cephalometric analysis showed a balanced cephalometric values (Table **10.1**) while frontal cephalometric analysis showed chin deviation to the patient's right side. CBCT sagittal screen shows lingual tipping of the crowns as posterior teeth in cross bite and the roots are almost out of the buccal plate of bone.

Treatment Objectives

In order to correct the patient's facial asymmetry, it would be easy to perform by fixing the unilateral posterior cross bite that would be needed to be corrected by uncontrolled tipping. Uncontrolled tipping is required in this case to move the crowns of the upper right posterior teeth buccally and the roots palatally. This palatal root movement is required to move the roots back into maxillary alveolar cancellous bone. It was hypothesized that eliminating dental interference due to the cross bite of the upper right lateral incisor would eliminate the functional shift and consequently correct the patient's facial asymmetry.

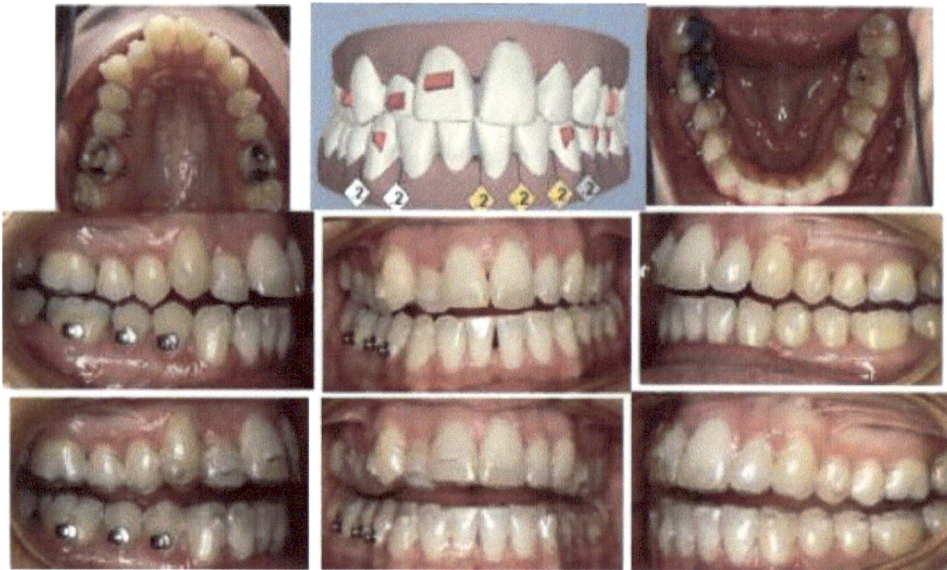

Fig. (10.3). Buttons were inserted for cross bite elastics and occlusal attachments on lower right first and second molars to eliminate occlusal interference can be seen (top right photo). It also can be seen that the patient's midlines are now coordinated.

Treatment Plan

Treatment planning included clear aligners and cross bite elastics from lower first molar on the buccal surface to the palatal surface of the upper first molar and right premolars. In order to facilitate treatment, occlusal bite clearance attachments were prescribed on the lower right first and second molars (Fig. **10.3**). Patient was fitted with 19 aligners. From day one, cross bite elastics (3/16" that produce 3.5 ounces of force) were recommended and the patient was instructed to wear these elastics every day all the time when the aligners were worn.

Treatment Progress

At stage 7 out of 19, patients midlines were already corrected, patient's facial asymmetry was improved and patient's right posterior cross bite was improved. Figure 64 compares before and stage 7 progresses. After 6 months, (total 19 trays with no refinement), the patient was completely finished treatment with cross bite improved and facial asymmetry improved (Fig. **10.4**).

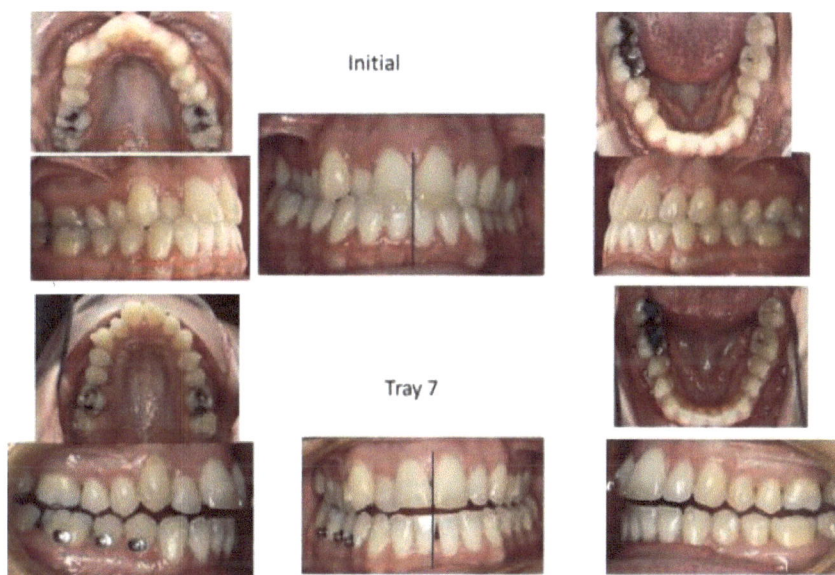

Fig. (10.4). Comparison before and after stage 7/19.

Patient was informed by her dentist that upper right lateral incisor, although cross bite was improved, it doesn't have adequate torque (Fig. **10.5**). When the patient presented with this concern, the patient was informed that there is no enough labial bone to move the root of that lateral incisor labialy to provide adequate torque and option of bone graft was presented. Patient understood the option and declined periodontal surgery.

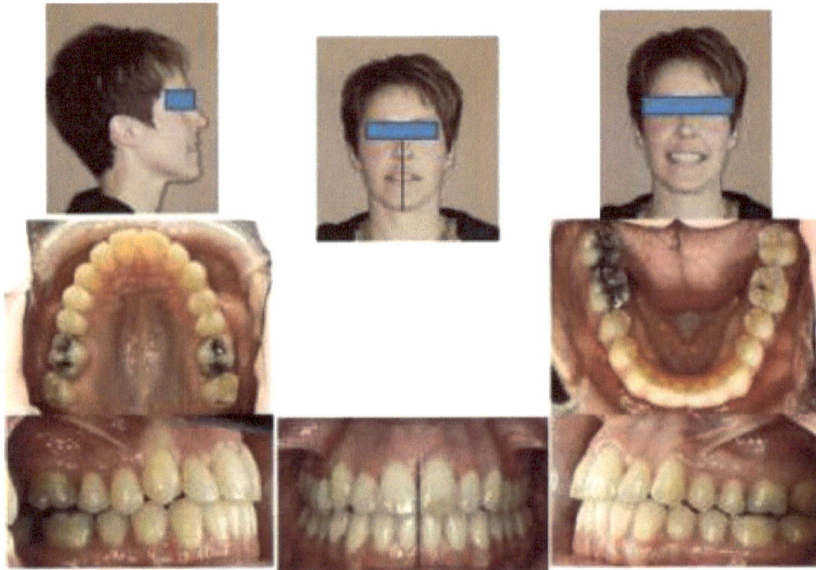

Fig. (10.5). Final records after 6 months treatment (stage 19). It can be seen that patient's face asymmetry is improved and cross bites were improved as well.

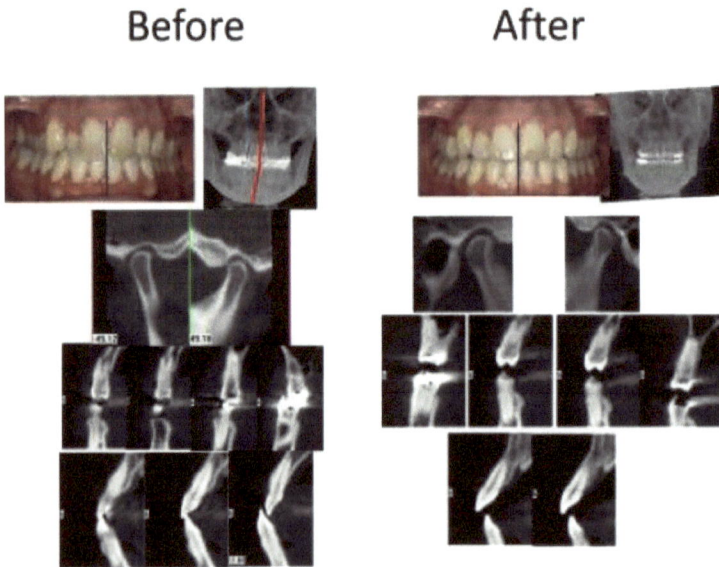

Fig. (10.6). Before and after Tomograms and sagittal screens as well as frontal cephalometric radiographs. It can be seen that condyles are well seated after treatment as well as right posterior teeth that were in cross bite are now well positioned within the alveolar bone.

Fig. (**10.6**) shows CBCT generated tomograms and sagittal screen showing that the posterior teeth are located within the alveolar bone with no roots out of the buccal cortical plate of bone. Fig. (**10.7**) shows superimposition of before and after frontal Cephalometric radiographs.

The patient was fitted with four Vivera retainers (Invisalign retainers) to be worn 24/7 for a year and night time afterwards.

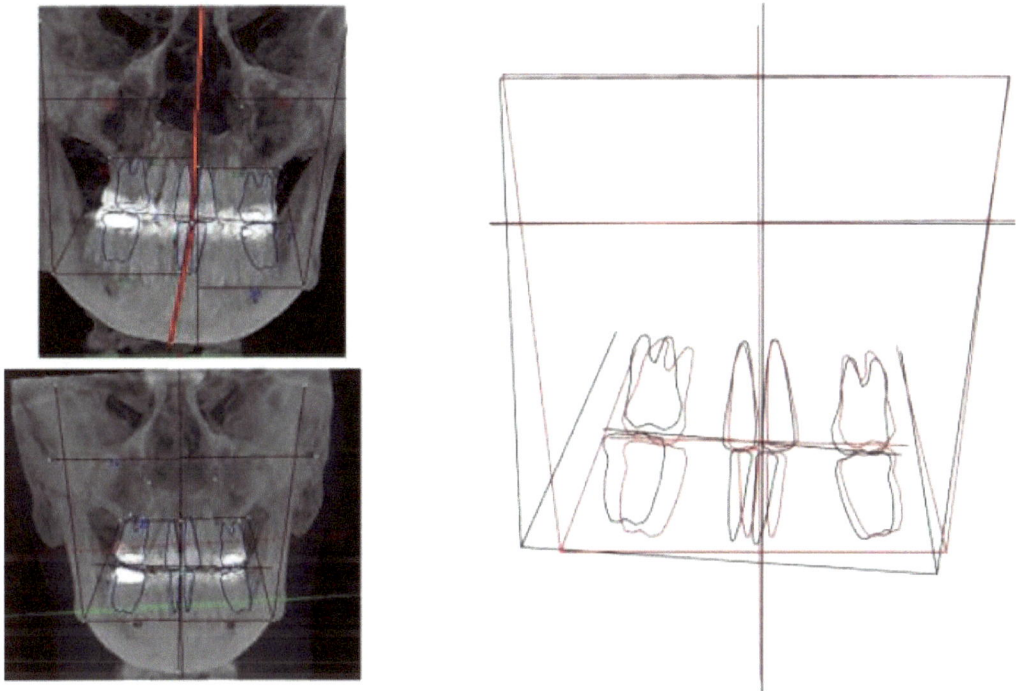

Fig. (10.7). Frontal cephalometric superimposition showing lateral shift (black) and corrected molars and mandible after treatment (red).

Table 10.1. PA cephalometric analysis of before and after treatment.

		Initial	After	Difference
Dental	Molar Relation, Left (mm)	-0.8	0.3	1.1
	Molar Relation, Right (mm)	-3.8	1.7	5.5
	Intermolar Width, Lower (mm)	54	50.3	-3.7
	Intermolar Width, Upper (mm)	49.4	52.3	2.9
	Denture Midline Discrepancy (mm)	0.6	0.1	-0.5

(Table 10.1) contd.....

		Initial	After	Difference
	Occlusal Plane Tilt (°)	4.8	1.8	-3
Dental/Skeletal				0
	Lower Arch Midline - MSR (mm)	-1.7	0.4	2.1
	Upper Arch Midline - MSR (mm)	-0.8	0.6	1.4
	Molar to Jaw, Left (mm)	7.4	7.3	-0.1
	Molar to Jaw, Right (mm)	8.3	6.8	-1.5
Skeletal				
	Frontal Convexity, Left (mm)	14	15.8	1.8
	Frontal Convexity, Right (mm)	21.3	20.2	-1.1
	GA - MSR (mm)	48.9	40.4	-8.5
	AG - MSR (mm)	35.9	38.3	2.4
	J - MSR, Left (mm)	28.4	28.2	-0.2
	J - MSR, Right (mm)	29.5	24.8	-4.7
	A - Me - MSR (°)	-7.6	-1.3	6.3
	Porion - MSR, Left (mm)	54.7	55.8	1.1
	Porion - MSR, Right (mm)	55.5	54.2	-1.3
	Nasal Width (mm)	28.8	27.2	-1.6

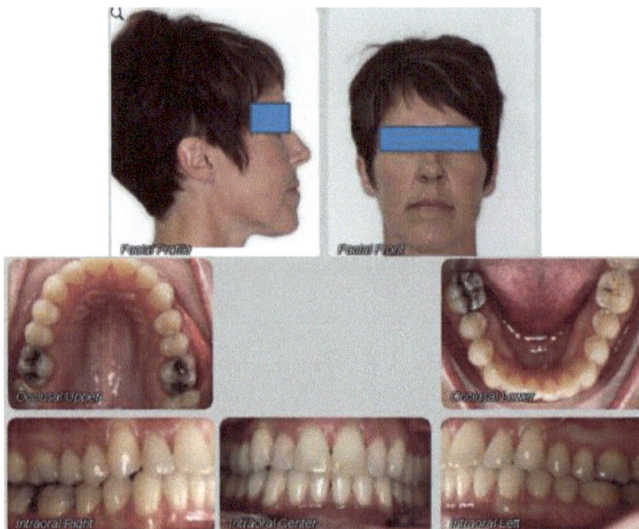

Fig. (10.8). Clinical photographs of the patient showing stable occlusion after two years of finishing the treatment and patient is wearing retainers at night time now after the first year in retention when the retainers were worn full time.

Retention photographs were taken 2 year after finishing the treatment and showed that the final treatment is stable (Fig. **10.8**). Patient was informed to continue wearing the retainers at night time for ever.

DISCUSSION

It is a common practice for adult patients with facial asymmetry to be candidates for surgical orthodontics. It is believed that a long standing facial asymmetry due to functional shift can lead to remodeling in the glenoid fossa and consequently surgical orthodontics is usually recommended in such cases. Tomogram is essential to diagnose whether there is a functional shift or not. The initial tomograms confirmed functional shift of the patient's mandible by differences in the anterior and posterior disc spaces between both right and left tomograms. This is in agreement with previous reports that confirmed different mandibular condylar positions before and after treatment [1, 4, 7, 8]. Although the patient has a slight constricted maxilla and this treatment involved buccal tipping of upper posterior teeth, this palatal root tipping moved the roots back lingually into maxillary alveolar cancellous bone. Although buccal tipping of the upper molars might be perceived as a compensation of the maxillary skeletal deficiency, in this case, this tooth movement helped moving the roots of the upper right posterior teeth from before treatment, that were almost out of the buccal cortical plate of bone, back into alveolar bone. The simple treatment in this case seems to have normalized right molar relationship, upper and lower intermolar widths and occlusal plane tilt.

Lateral cephalometric analyses of before and after treatment show improvement of the patient skeletal apical base relationship (ANB). However, the treatment results in our case disagree with previous reports that persistent functional shift due to posterior cross bite is only treated by orthognathic surgery. CBCT-generated tomograms with lower radiation dose can provide more insights into the position of condyles in cases with unilateral posterior crossbite that can lead to functional shift in adults which can be easily treated by simple upper arch expansion and coordination with lower dental arch without the need for surgical orthodontics.

SUMMARY AND RECOMMENDATION

In summary, facial asymmetry can be treated by clear aligners without the need for orthognathic surgery as long as proper diagnosis and treatment planning is performed. It can be seen that CBCT is crucial in diagnosis such cases in order to eliminate or minimize major surgeries.

REFERENCES

[1] Akahane Y, Deguchi T, Hunt NP. Morphology of the temporomandibular joint in skeletal class iii symmetrical and asymmetrical cases: a study by cephalometric laminography. J Orthod 2001; 28(2): 119-28.
[http://dx.doi.org/10.1093/ortho/28.2.119] [PMID: 11395526]

[2] Fuentes MA, Opperman LA, Buschang P, Bellinger LL, Carlson DS, Hinton RJ. Lateral functional shift of the mandible: Part I. Effects on condylar cartilage thickness and proliferation. Am J Orthod Dentofacial Orthop 2003; 123(2): 153-9.
[http://dx.doi.org/10.1067/mod.2003.5] [PMID: 12594421]

[3] Fuentes MA, Opperman LA, Buschang P, Bellinger LL, Carlson DS, Hinton RJ. Lateral functional shift of the mandible: Part II. Effects on gene expression in condylar cartilage. Am J Orthod Dentofacial Orthop 2003; 123(2): 160-6.
[http://dx.doi.org/10.1067/mod.2003.6] [PMID: 12594422]

[4] Hesse KL, Artun J, Joondeph DR, Kennedy DB. Changes in condylar postition and occlusion associated with maxillary expansion for correction of functional unilateral posterior crossbite. Am J Orthod Dentofacial Orthop 1997; 111(4): 410-8.
[http://dx.doi.org/10.1016/S0889-5406(97)80023-6] [PMID: 9109586]

[5] Kecik D, Kocadereli I, Saatci I. Evaluation of the treatment changes of functional posterior crossbite in the mixed dentition. Am J Orthod Dentofacial Orthop 2007; 131(2): 202-15.
[http://dx.doi.org/10.1016/j.ajodo.2005.03.030] [PMID: 17276861]

[6] Kilic N, Kiki A, Oktay H. Condylar asymmetry in unilateral posterior crossbite patients. Am J Orthod Dentofacial Orthop 2008; 133(3): 382-7.
[http://dx.doi.org/10.1016/j.ajodo.2006.04.041] [PMID: 18331937]

[7] Lam PH, Sadowsky C, Omerza F. Mandibular asymmetry and condylar position in children with unilateral posterior crossbite. Am J Orthod Dentofacial Orthop 1999; 115(5): 569-75.
[http://dx.doi.org/10.1016/S0889-5406(99)70282-9] [PMID: 10229892]

[8] O'Byrn BL, Sadowsky C, Schneider B, BeGole EA. An evaluation of mandibular asymmetry in adults with unilateral posterior crossbite. Am J Orthod Dentofacial Orthop 1995; 107(4): 394-400.
[http://dx.doi.org/10.1016/S0889-5406(95)70092-7] [PMID: 7709904]

[9] Sato C, Muramoto T, Soma K. Functional lateral deviation of the mandible and its positional recovery on the rat condylar cartilage during the growth period. Angle Orthod 2006; 76(4): 591-7.
[PMID: 16808564]

[10]   Wong CA, Sinclair PM, Keim RG, Kennedy DB. Arch dimension changes from successful slow maxillary expansion of unilateral posterior crossbite. Angle Orthod 2011; 81(4): 616-23.
[http://dx.doi.org/10.2319/072210-429.1] [PMID: 21306221]

CHAPTER 11

Treatment of Challenging Cases Using Clear Aligners

Abstract: Limitations of using clear aligners include noncompliance and compromised/fair oral hygiene. Rotational tooth movement also could be a challenge. Small thin teeth are also hard to move. The following chapter will discuss these limitations and possible strategies to manage these limitations.

Keywords: Case selection, Challenging tooth movement, Clear aligners, Compliance, Decalcification, Limitations, Outcomes, Relapse, Retention, Prognosis.

In a paper published in 2007, clinical limitations of clear aligners, especially Invisalign were presented [1]. In this paper, the authors outlined some malocclusions that he outlined as not candidates for clear aligners treatment. These conditions are 1) crowding and spacing over 5 mm; 2) skeletal anterior-posterior discrepancies of more than 2 mm (as measured by discrepancies in cuspid relationships); 3) centric-relation and centric-occlusion discrepancies; 4) severely rotated teeth (more than 20 degrees); 5) open bites (anterior and posterior) that need to be closed; 6) extrusion of teeth; 7) severely tipped teeth (more than 45 degrees); 8) teeth with short clinical crowns; and 9) arches with multiple missing teeth. Although these conditions might have been difficult to treat in 2007 not all of them are not candidates for clear aligners.

You can see in this book that some difficult cases like severe apical base discrepancies (skeletal Class II and class III) are treated successfully in this book. Also, severely tipped teeth (Case 4 in class II chapter) is treated within a year. Also, cases with centric-relation and centric-occlusion discrepancies can be treat-

Tarek El-Bialy, Donna Galante & Sam Daher

ed now with clear aligners (Facial asymmetric, Chapter 10 of this book). Although, there are no open bite cases presented in this book but there have been many reports in the literature about effective treatment of open bite cases with clear aligners [2 - 7].

In recent presentation at Invisalign Summit for orthodontists in November 2012, it was declared to all attendees that any orthodontic case can be treated by clear aligners. In this book chapter, two cases are presented highlighting the limitations of clear aligners.

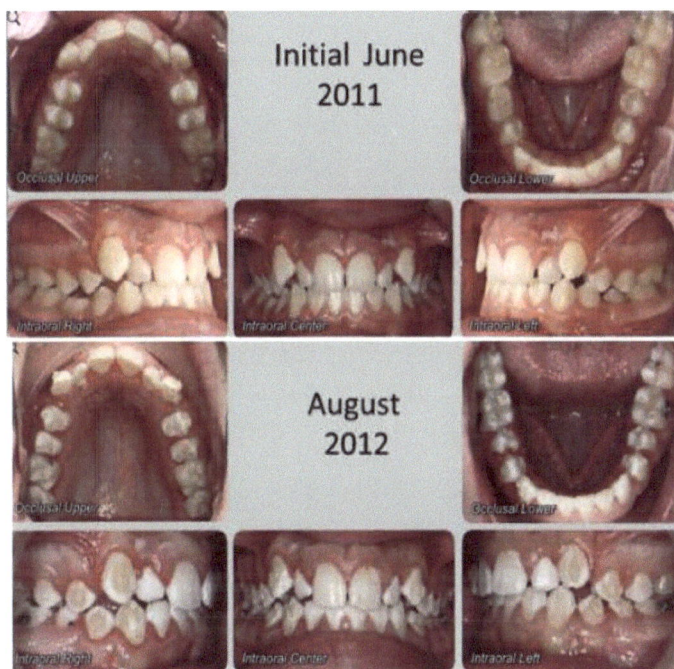

Fig. (11.1). The top above intraoral photos revealed fair oral hygiene starting in June 2011. Progress photos (bottom raw) show severe hypo-mineralization after a one year treatment and hypertrophic gingival growth.

Case 1

This twelve-year old male presented in June 2011 with a chief complain that he had moderate to minimum crowded upper and lower teeth that required them to be treated. The patient presented initially with fair oral hygiene that was instructed to improve during the course of treatment. After one year of Invisalign wear, the patient developed a severe hypocalcification (Fig. **11.1**). The dentist was in a position to stop the treatment until remineralization occurs. After discussion with the patient, parents and the dentist, the patient continued to wear the clear aligners and was instructed to us the clear aligners as fluoride. Clinical follow up revealed partial remineralization however not fully recovered.

This could be attributed to the fact that clear aligners may be working as microbial/plaque incubator if the patient does not maintain excellent oral hygiene. Part of this problem is that some patients cannot clean the aligners from inside as they are supposed to. Clear instructions to the patients to make sure that they should keep the aligners clear that the patients can see through them. If the aligners start to be cloudy, it is not advisable to use them until the patient cleans them thoroughly.

Case 2

This is a 45-year-old female who presented to the orthodontic clinic with a complaint of relapsed crowded teeth after initial orthodontic treatment. She had minimum upper and lower minimum dental crowding (Fig. **11.2**). Patient was given different treatment options including clear braces metal braces and she requested clear aligners. After consultation and discussing the pros and cons of each technique, the patient was insistent to have clear aligners for her treatment.

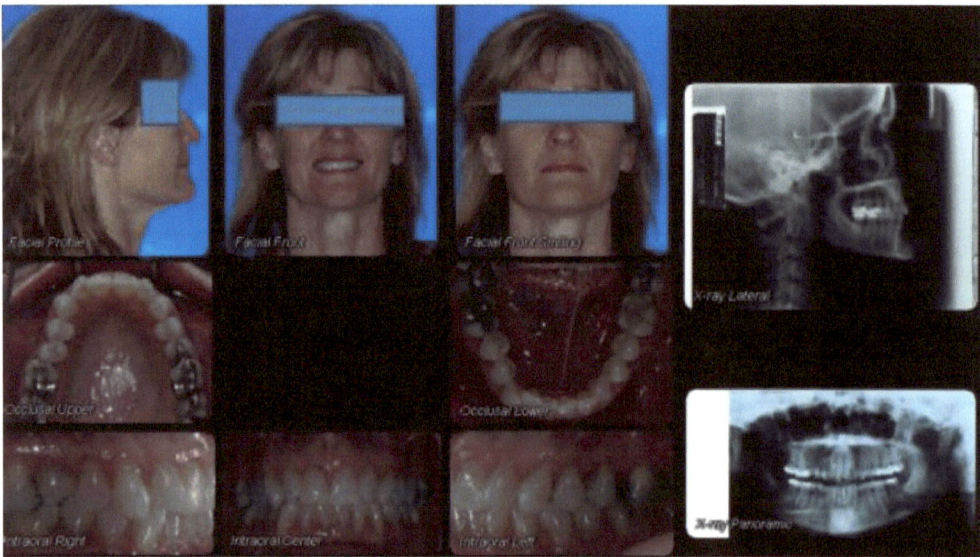

Fig. (11.2). Initial records of the 45-year old female.

The patient was initially fitted with 22 aligners in December 2007 that he was instructed to wear those aligners 20-22 hours/day and change them every two weeks. After 48 weeks, there was improvement in incisors alignment however results were not fully satisfactory to the patient (Fig. **11.3**).

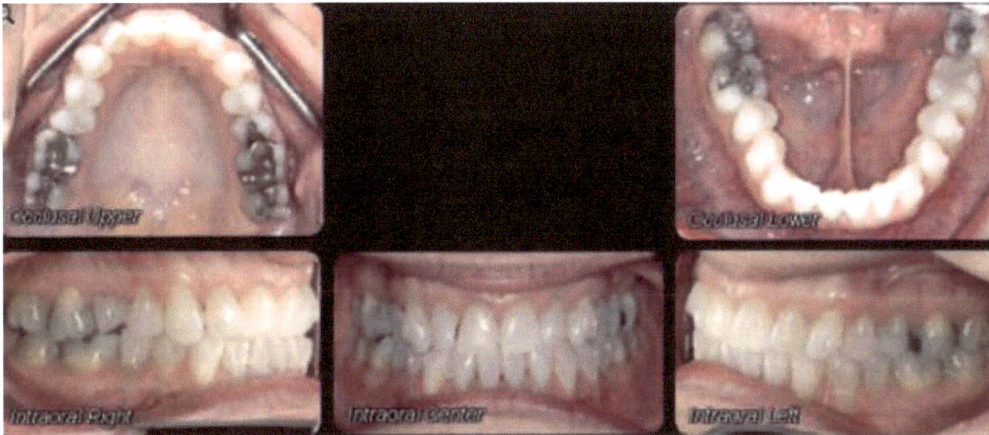

Fig. (11.3). Clinical records after the first set of aligners and they were used for refinement.

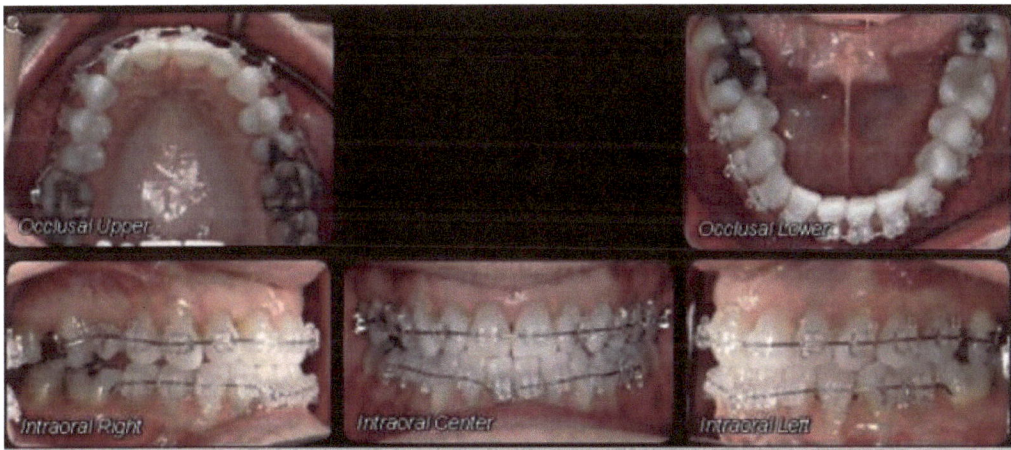

Fig. (11.4). Clinical records after refinement in June 2009 (Day of bonding).

The patient was fitted with another set of 18 refinement aligners. After 36 weeks, the patient was not fully satisfied and requested full fixed clear braces that were inserted in June 2009 (Fig. **11.4**). After four months, the patient was satisfied with the results and deboned in October 2009 (Fig. **11.5**).

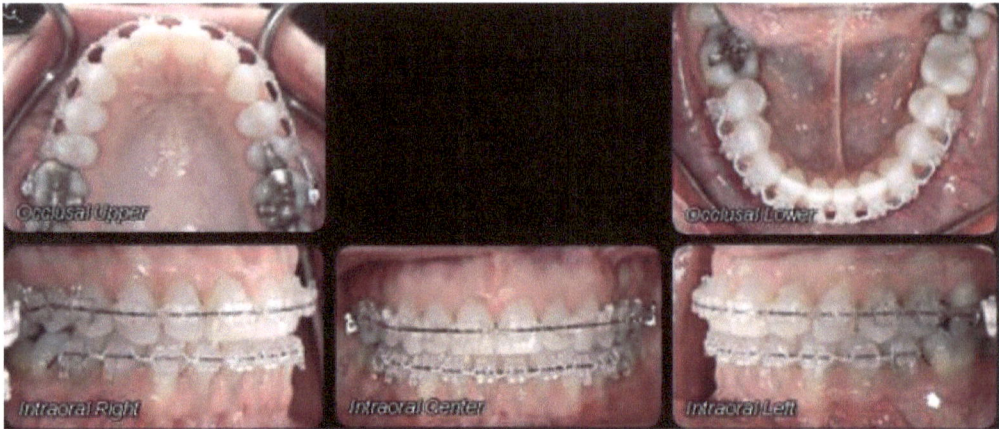

Fig. (11.5). Clinical records before deboning in October 2009.

Critical Analysis of the Cases

Old clear aligners' materials might not be effective in producing effective tooth movement which has been claimed recently by Align technology. Lateral incisors have been reported to be the most difficult teeth to align due to the fact that their anatomy is small and difficult to be grasped by clear aligners. New development in the technology and new materials might be more flexible to grasp teeth and consequently move them. It is to be noted that at the current time, Invisalign or clear aligners in general might not be the best option for all cases, especially non-compliant patients. Future development of the technique and materials might make it suitable for difficult cases.

REFERENCES

[1]   Phan X, Ling PH. Clinical limitations of Invisalign. J Can Dent Assoc 2007; 73(3): 263-6.
      [PMID: 17439714]

[2]   Boyd RL. Complex orthodontic treatment using a new protocol for the Invisalign appliance. J Clin Orthod 2007; 41(9): 525-47.
      [PMID: 17921600]

[3]   Womack WR, Ahn JH, Ammari Z, Castillo A. A new approach to correction of crowding. Am J Orthod Dentofacial Orthop 2002; 122(3): 310-6.
      [http://dx.doi.org/10.1067/mod.2002.127477] [PMID: 12226614]

[4]   Clements KM, Bollen AM, Huang G, King G, Hujoel P, Ma T. Activation time and material stiffness of sequential removable orthodontic appliances. Part 2: Dental improvements. Am J Orthod Dentofacial Orthop 2003; 124(5): 502-8.

[http://dx.doi.org/10.1016/S0889-5406(03)00577-8] [PMID: 14614416]

[5]   Levrini L, Tettamanti L, Macchi A, Tagliabue A, Caprioglio A. Invisalign teen for thumb-sucking management. A case report. Eur J Paediatr Dent 2012; 13(2): 155-8.
[PMID: 22762181]

[6]   Harnick DJ. Using clear aligner therapy to correct malocclusion with crowding and an open bite. Gen Dent 2012; 60(3): 218-23.
[PMID: 22623461]

[7]   Schupp W, Haubrich J, Neumann I. Treatment of anterior open bite with the Invisalign system. J Clin Orthod 2010; 44(8): 501-7.
[PMID: 21105589]

CHAPTER 12

Surgical Orthodontics Treatment with Invisalign

Abstract: Surgical orthodontic treatment is usually required in cases having severe skeletal mal-relationships and malocclusion that cannot be resolved solely by orthodontic treatment. In managing surgical orthodontic cases, pre-surgical orthodontic treatment usually aims at coordinating both dental arches, eliminating dental compensation due to the skeletal mal-relationship if present and to eliminate any dental interferences once dental arches are occluding together after the skeletal mal-relationship is corrected by surgical intervention. Post-surgical orthodontic treatment usually aims at finishing and detailing dental arch relationships and ensure that no interferences exist. Traditionally, pre-surgical and post-surgical orthodontic treatments are usually achieved by regular fixed orthodontic appliances and pre-surgical orthodontics usually require having the patients wearing heavy archwires in order to be used for inter-maxillary fixation after surgery. The introduction of clear aligners in surgical orthodontics was initially somehow not well-received by orthodontists and oral surgeons due to the fact that rigid archwires are needed before surgery and clear aligners may have limitations on what can be done in terms of preparing cases with skeletal mal-relationships for orthognathic surgeries. The present chapter will shed the light on surgical orthodontic cases that were treated solely by clear aligners before and after orthognathic surgeries as well as describe steps in management of such cases using clear aligners.

Keywords: Clear aligners, Decompensation, Diagnosis, Orthodontics, Post-surgical, Pre-surgical, Stability, Surgical orthodontics, Temporary anchorage devices, Treatment planning.

INTRODUCTION

Surgical orthodontic correction of dentofacial deformities including jaw mal-relationship aims to improve facial aesthetic and function in these cases [1]. A successful outcome of orthognathic surgery depends on the planning and execut-

Tarek El-Bialy, Donna Galante & Sam Daher

ion of orthodontic and surgical techniques [2 - 5]. Surgical orthodontic planning involves model surgery, traditional cephalometric prediction as well as photographic prediction or utilization of computerized cephalometric/photo-graphic predictions [6, 7]. Model surgical prediction suffers from potential errors including model mounting of jaw relationship by face bow/bite transfer. In complex cases, dental compensation and crowding may necessitate extraction of teeth. In class II skeletal cases when extraction is required for decompensation and relieving crowding is needed, the extraction pattern usually involves lower first premolars and upper second premolars. The reverse pattern is usually the case in severe skeletal class III. However, in many cases where dental compensation is not too severe, or when crowding is not moderate or severe, extraction may not be necessary for pre-surgical orthodontics phase. Many cases can be treated pre-surgically by arch development (expansion) and incisors torque as well as interproximal reduction.

Align technology uses a digital diagnostic set up, using Clincheck® software, that allows the clinician to plan and predict tooth alignment, dental arch relationships, as well as viewing dental occlusion from different aspects that are normally hard to see or evaluate using plaster models. In addition, it helps clinicians with planning the treatment as well as mitigating dental interferences before they occur.

Case 1

This is a 27 year-old female that was presented with a chief complaint that she had overbite and a small chin. Clinical examination and clinical records (Figs. **12.1** & **12.2**) revealed the following findings:

1. Convex profile with recessive chin and relatively large nose and increased nasolabial angle.
2. Class II skeletal and dental relationships due to mandibular retrognathism
3. ANB angle = 6.6°
4. Overjet = 8 mm and overbite is 80%
5. Increased curve of Spee
6. Minimum crowding of the upper arch that was narrow (tapered) and no

crowding in the lower dental arch.

7. Wisdom teeth were missing and no major dental anomalies.

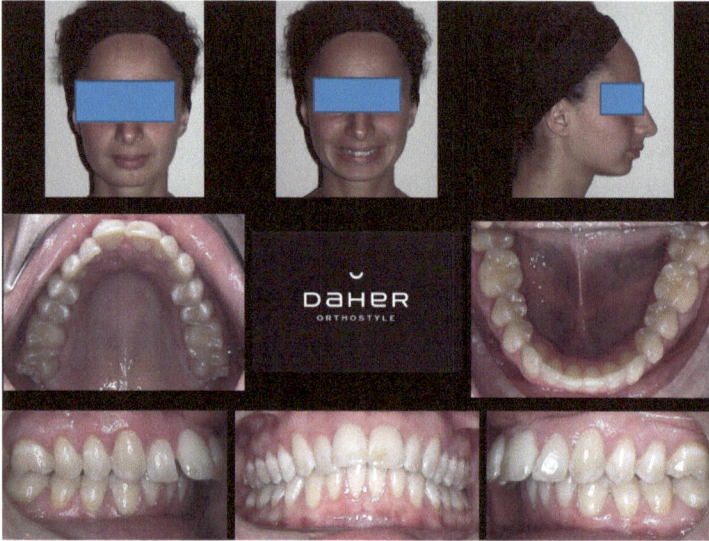

Fig. (12.1). Initial clinical records of patient #1. Extraoral photos show patient had a convex profile due to recessive chin and relatively large nose. Class II division 1 malocclusion with increased curve of Spee.

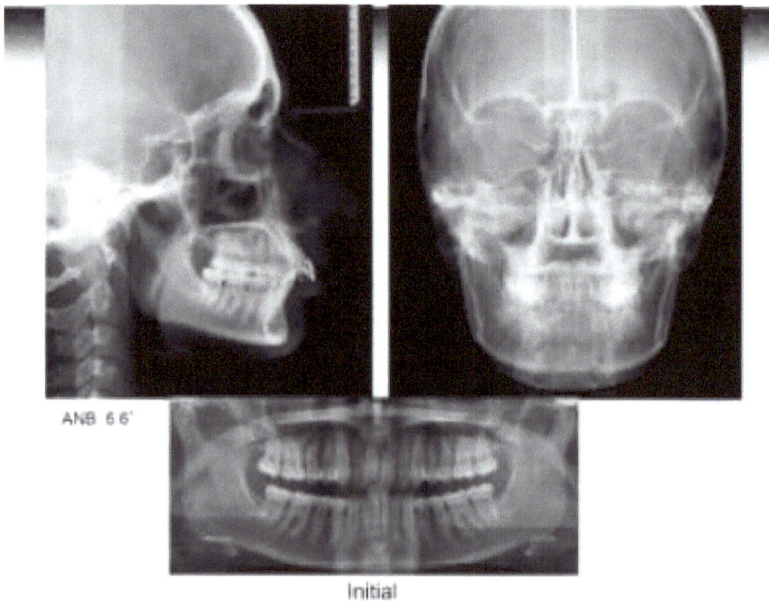

Fig. (12.2). Initial radiographs showing skeletal Class II relation.

Treatment Objectives

1. Improve patient's profile by advancing her mandible *via* bilateral sagittal split osteotomy (BSSO) and using temporary anchorage devices (TADs) for elastic wear.
2. Improve the patient's occlusion to full class I molars and canines
3. Improve patient's overjet and curve of Spee.
4. Relieve crowding.

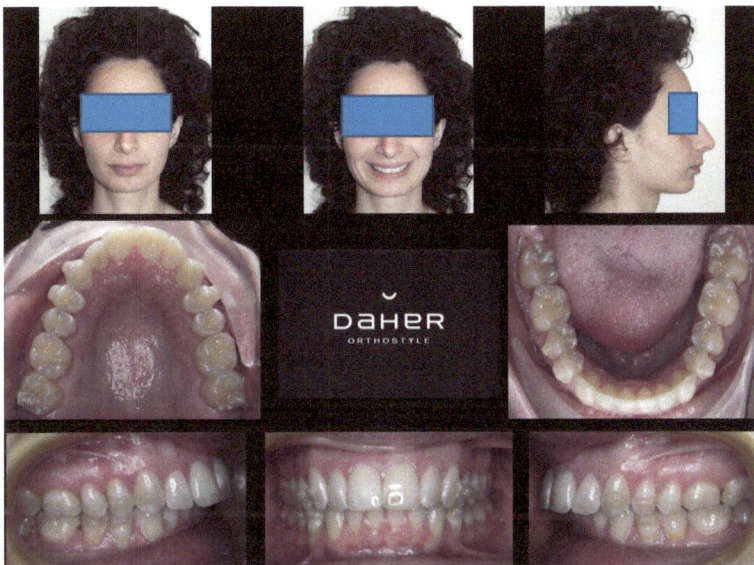

Fig. (12.3). Pre-surgical records showing upper arch expansion and relieve of the patient's upper crowding.

Treatment Progress

1. Patient had pre-surgical orthodontics utilizing Invisalign that included 21 upper and 22 lower aligners.
2. Curve of Spee was improved by intruding lower incisors and extruding lower premolars by using horizontal attachments on the lower premolars.
3. Pre-surgical records (Fig. **12.3**) show proper upper incisors alignment, upper arch was expanded to allow for mandibular forward positioning by BSSO.
4. Immediate post-surgical records (Fig. **12.4** and **12.5**) show improvement of the patient's profile, chin prominence, class I molars and canines and inter-maxillary fixation was performed using mini-screws (four in each arch for

inter-maxillary elastics) (Fig. **12.6**).

5. According to the recommendation by Dr. Daher, elastics protocol post-surgery was worn by the patient as follows:

   a. Elastics: Upper to Lower TAD's:

   b. Size: 5/16" (8mm), 3 oz (100 grams), full-time

   c. 2-3 weeks in total

   d. Wear U & L aligners full-time

6. Reasons for elastics are described by Proffit [8] as follows: "Light vertical elastics are needed initially, not so much for the tooth movement but to override proprioceptive impulses from the teeth that otherwise would cause the patient to seek a new position of maximum intercuspation" [8].

7. The duration for 2-3 weeks post-surgery of elastics wear has been reported by Proffit [9] to allow for early function and early finishing of the case orthodontically.

8. Post-surgical orthodontic treatment involves continuous level of the curve of Spee, utilizing buttons bonded to the lower premolars and molars that can be extruded using vertical elastics to the upper TADs (Figs. **12.7-12.9**).

9. Settling posterior occlusion can also be achieved by adding buccal buttons to the upper molars for vertical posterior elastics between buttons bonded to upper and lower posterior teeth (Fig. **12.10**).

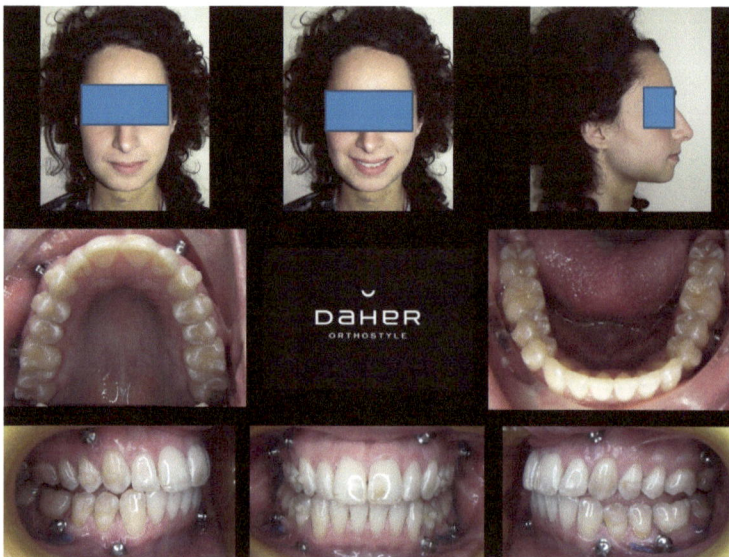

Fig. (12.4). Patient's photographs at 11th day post-surgery showing TADs in place for posterior teeth settling.

Post-Surgery cephalometric
and panoramic radiographs

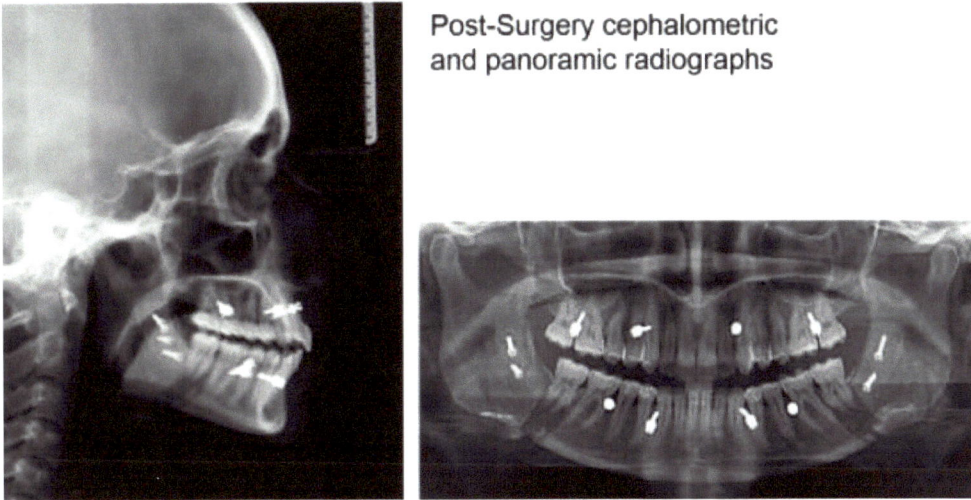

Fig. (12.5). Post-surgical radiographs showing correction of the skeletal Class II relation.

Temporary Anchorage Device (TAD)

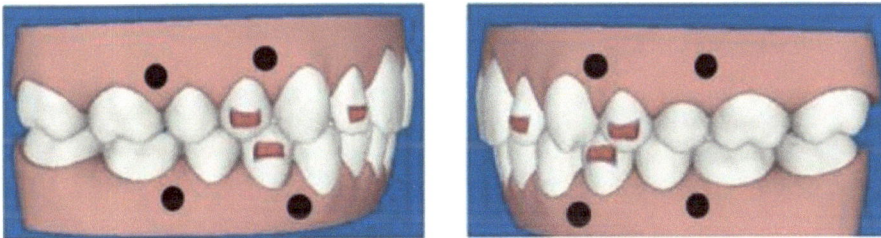

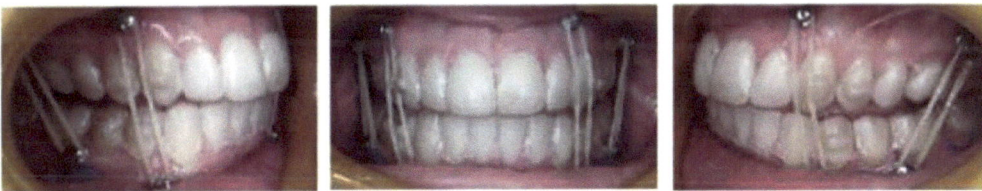

11 days post-Sx

Fig. (12.6). Intraoral photographs and clincheck showing TADS and elastic pattern.

10. Care should be taken not to overdo elastics wear in this pattern. It should be

noted that applying vertical elastics from the buccal surface can rotate upper and lower molars' crowns lingually as the lines of action of these forces are buccal to the center of resistances of upper and lower posterior teeth and this leads to a moment that tends to rotate the posterior teeth crowns lingually. This may be advantageous in cases where upper and lower molars are tipped buccally either by pre-surgical orthodontic expansion or due to pre-existing position of these teeth uprighted. Applying the vertical elastics in these cases can provide normal torque of the posterior teeth as described by Andrews when he explained the need for lingual crown torque in adult normal occlusion [10]. If however a case shows normal posterior teeth crown angulation (torque), vertical elastics may be applied both buccally and lingually in order to maintain teeth axial inclination.

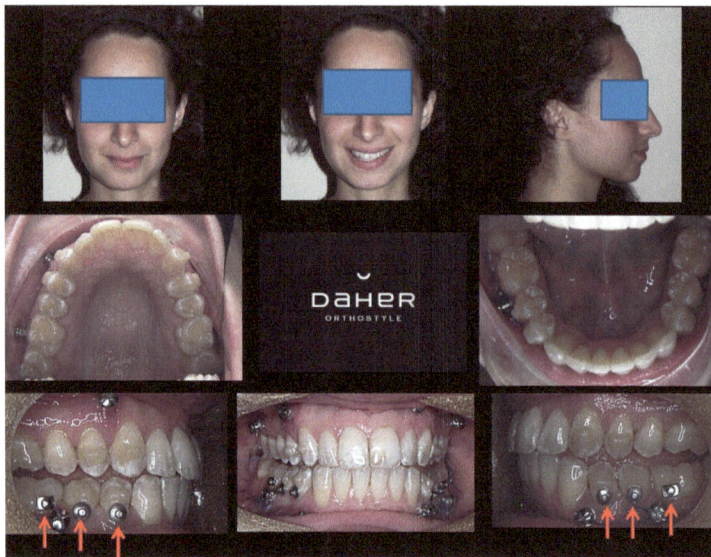

Fig. (12.7). Intraoral photographs showing buttons and TADs for lower premolar extrusion to level the curve of Spee.

11. It should also be noted that these buccal buttons attached to the teeth can be utilized to correct minor antero-posterior bite issues. For example, Fig. (**12.10**) shows how left side elastics are more vertical to allow for posterior teeth settling (right side) or have a class II component (left side).

12. Fig. (**12.11**) shows that the posterior teeth are settling using different types of elastics patterns.

13. Fig. (**12.12**) shows patient's final occlusion after 14 weeks of post-surgical Invisalign orthodontic treatment.

14. Fig. (**12.13**) shows the patient's profile before, while the patient is posturing forward after the treatment.

15. Fig. (**12.14**) shows the patient's cephalometric radiographs before and after surgery and indicates that the ANB angle reduced from 6.6° at the beginning to 3.9° after treatment.

16. Retention was prescribed as full time wear of retainers for a year and night time for the rest of the patient's life.

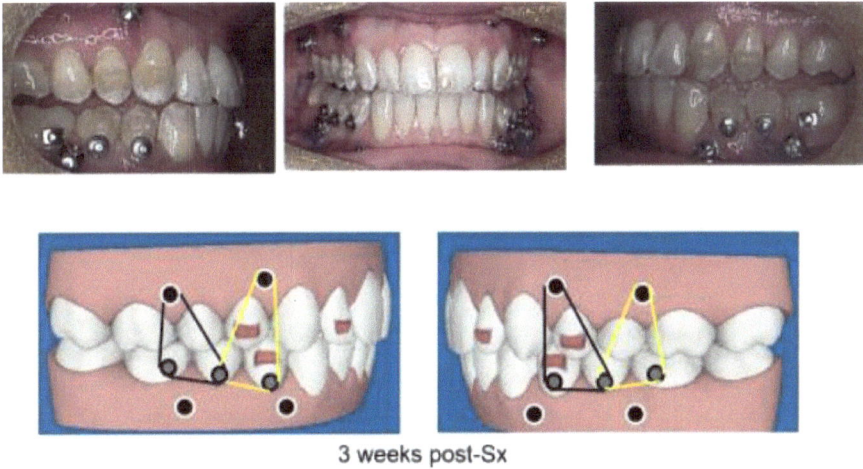

3 weeks post-Sx

Fig. (12.8). Intraoral photographs/clincheck showing elastic pattern to level the curve of Spee.

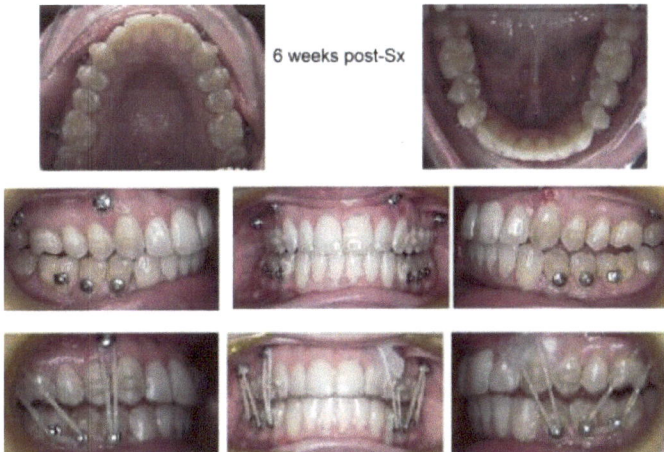

6 weeks post-Sx

Fig. (12.9). Intraoral photographs 6 weeks post-surgery showing elastic pattern to level the curve of Spee that has been improved.

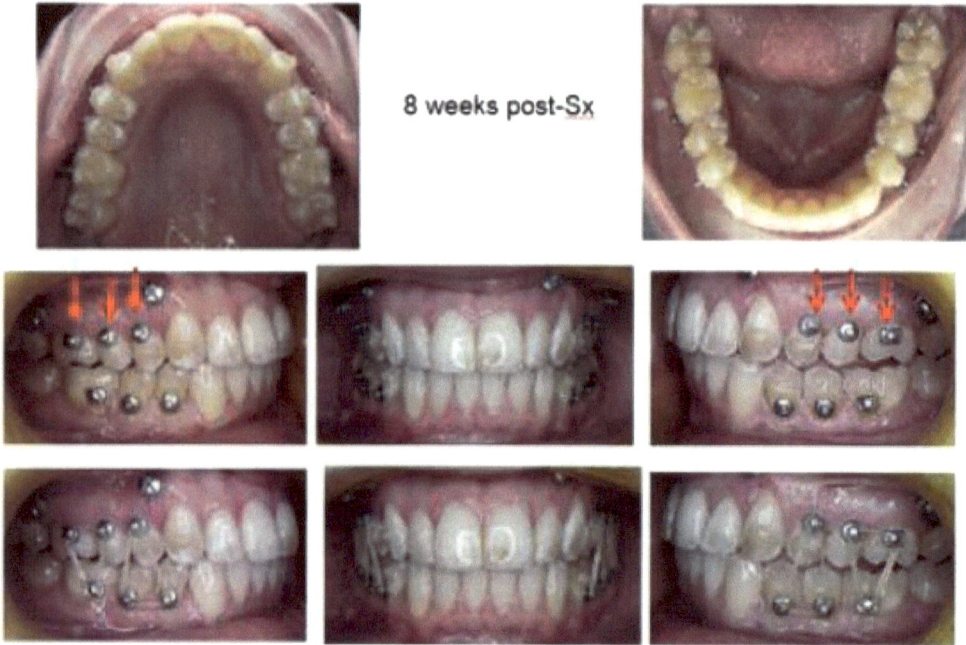

Fig. (12.10). Intraoral photographs 8 weeks post-surgery (Sx) showing elastic pattern to level the curve of Spee that has been improved and right premolars/molars are in contact with the upper posterior teeth.

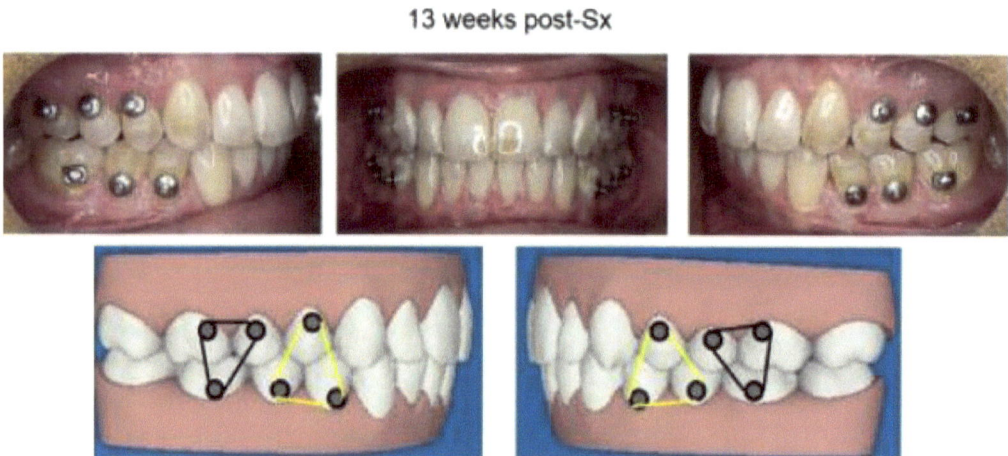

Fig. (12.11). Intraoral photographs /clincheck 13 weeks post-surgery showing elastic pattern to level the curve of Spee that has been improved and all right and left premolars/molars are in contact with the upper posterior teeth.

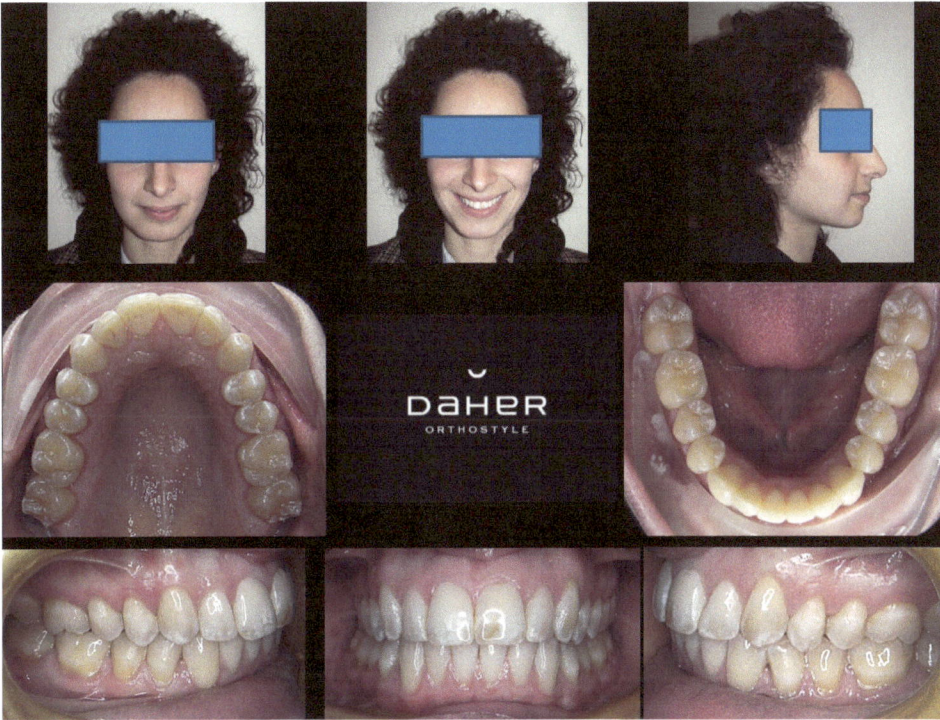

Fig. (12.12). Final clinical photographs 14 weeks post-surgery showing improved patient profile and maximum intercuspation as well as normal overbite and overjet.

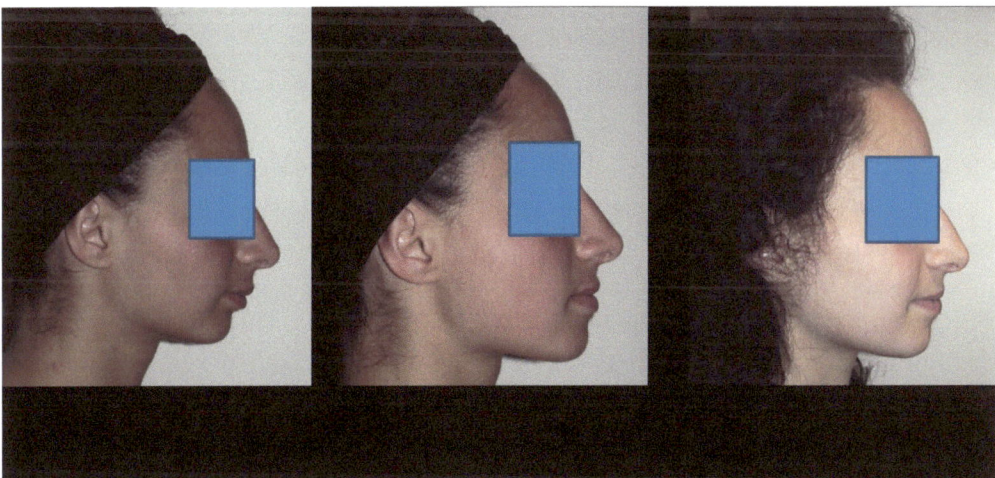

Fig. (12.13). Facial photographs of the patient's profiles, initial with mandibular forward posturing (simulating surgery) and final showing that surgical orthodontic treatment with Invisalign is predictable and simulating initial profile while the patient is posturing forward.

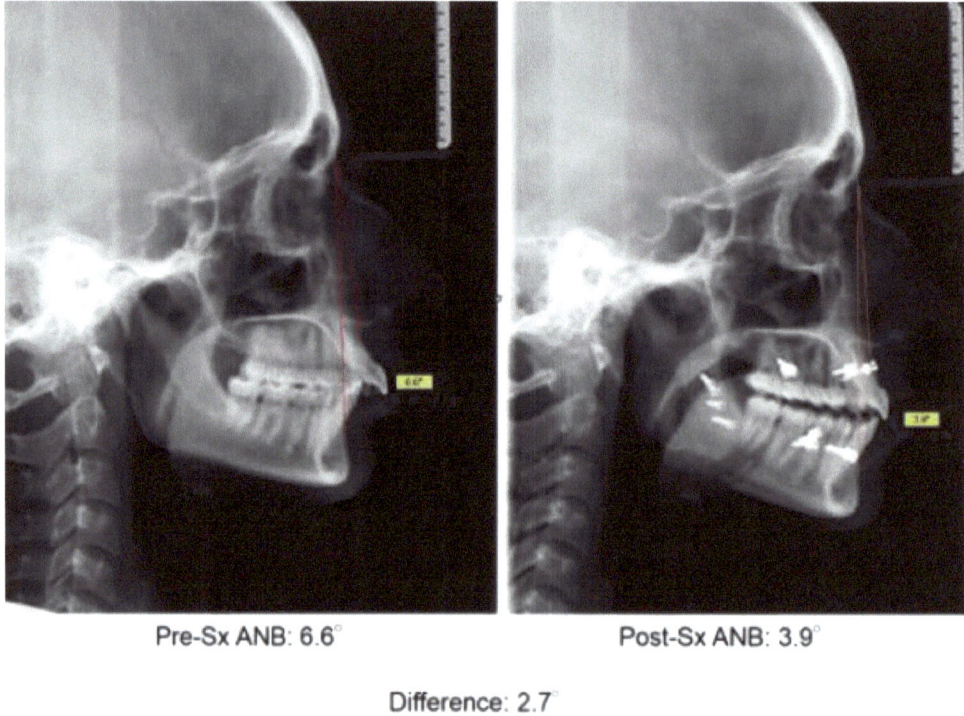

Pre-Sx ANB: 6.6°   Post-Sx ANB: 3.9°

Difference: 2.7°

Fig. (12.14). Comparison of patient's cephalometric radiographs before and after surgery.

Case Summary

Surgical orthodontic treatment of an adult case with skeletal class II due to mandibular deficiency with Invisalign and surgical mandibular advancement is predictable. Also, it has been observed that in surgical cases treated with Invisalign, surgical wound heals faster than surgical wound with regular orthodontic braces.

This might be attributed to the fact that oral hygiene is much improved with Invisalign as a removable appliance as compared to that with fixed orthodontic appliance [11]. Also, this might be attributed to the fact that similar plastic (Essix) to the ones used with Invisalign treatment has a piezoelectric effect that may have an added effect on tissue healing [12]. However, this property needs to be proven by future research on the plastic used by Invisalign system.

Case 2

This 25 year-old healthy female presented with a chief concern of increase overbite and sought fixing her esthetics. Also, she reported TMJ occasional click upon maximum opening and it is asymptomatic. Intraoral photos revealed Class II division 1 malocclusion with skeletal Class II due to mandibular retrognathism. Clinical examination revealed that she has incompetent lips with mentalis muscle strain as well as increased overjet (7 mm) and overbite which were found to be 50% (Fig. **12.15**). History and radiographic examination revealed that all her third molars were missing (Fig. **12.16**).

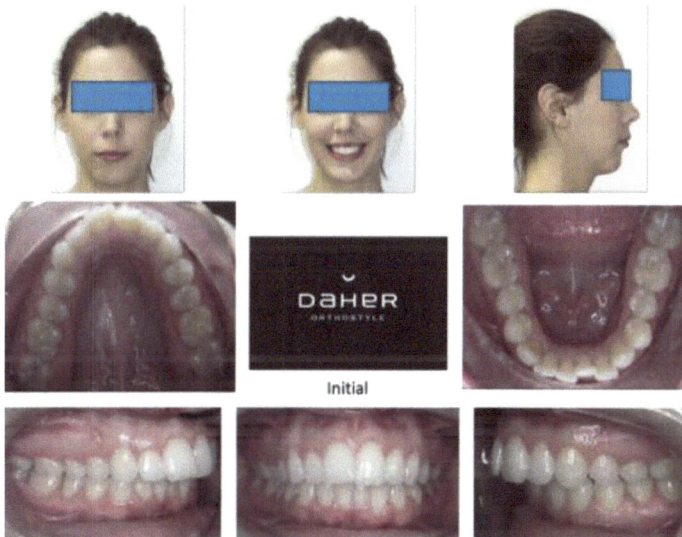

Fig. (12.15). Case 2 initial photos.

Treatment Objectives

1. Align upper and lower incisors;
2. Consultation for surgical mandibular advancement using bilateral sagittal split osteotomy;
3. Post-surgical orthodontic phase for detailing and provide maximum intercuspation;
4. Retention

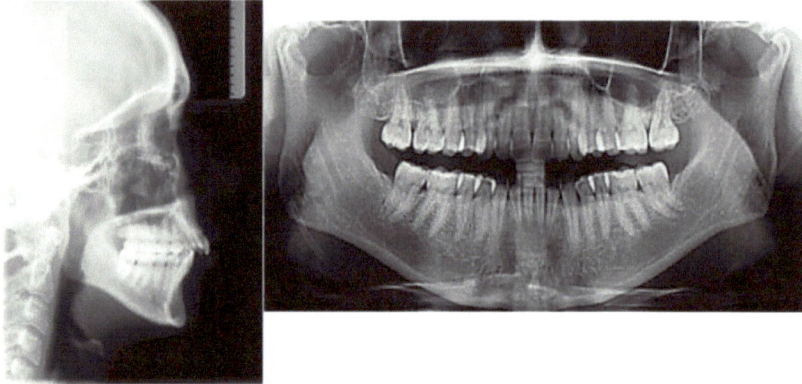

Fig. (12.16). Case 2 initial radiographs. Lateral cephalometric radiograph revealed skeletal class II relationship due to mandibular retrognathism.

Treatment Progress

Patient accepted the surgical orthodontic treatment and proceeded with initial leveling and alignment using Invisalign treatment (11 upper and lower aligners) for 6 months (Fig. **12.17**).

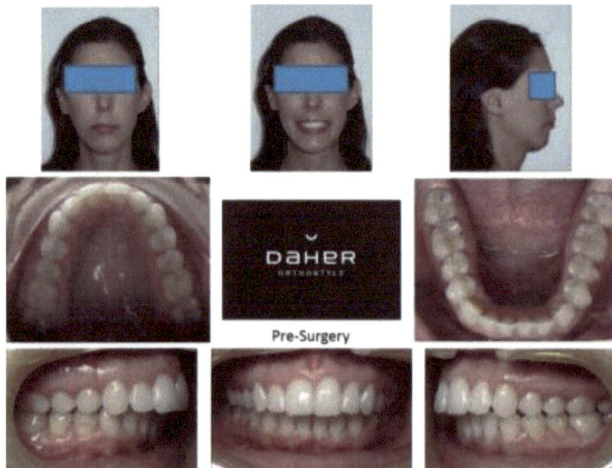

Fig. (12.17). Case 2, pre-surgical photos.

Surgical mandibular advancement commenced after the initial level and alignment utilizing bilateral sagittal split osteotomy with intermaxillary elastics as indicated in Case 1 (Figs. **12.18-12.20**). Post-surgery, patient underwent refinement including 8 upper and lower aligners to change every 10 days and this phase continued for 3 months (Fig. **12.21**). Total treatment time was 11 months then the patient was fitted with Vivera® retainers. (Fig. **12.22**) shows final clinical photos of the patient and (Figs. **12.23** and **12.24**) shows comparison between before and final photos.

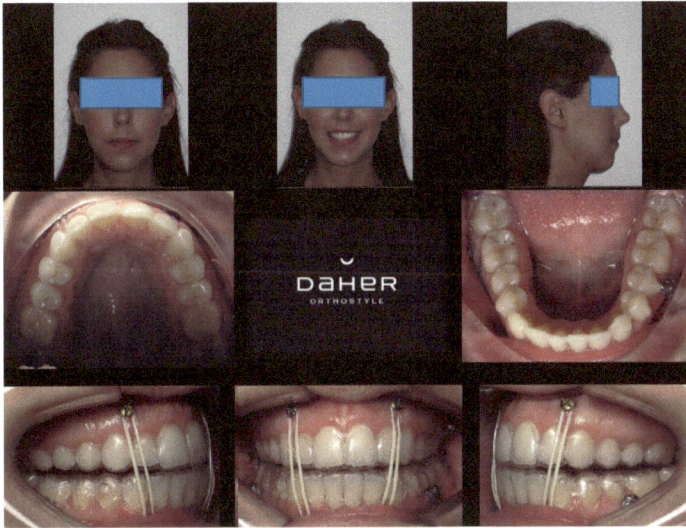

Fig. (12.18). Case 2, postsurgical photos showing intermaxillary elastics hooked to anterior and posterior TADs.

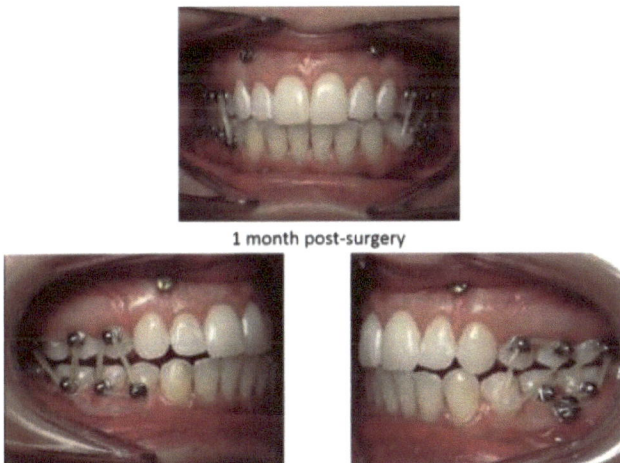

Fig. (12.19). Case 2, 1 month postsurgical intraoral photos showing intermaxillary elastics between posterior teeth for settling of the posterior teeth and closing posterior open bite.

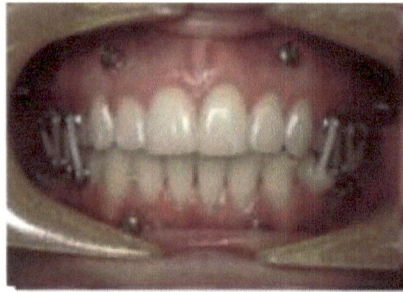

3 weeks of elastics

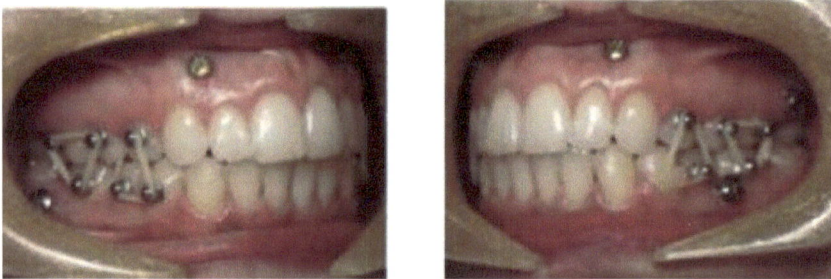

Fig. (12.20). Case 2, intraoral photos after three weeks of wearing posterior elastics showing closure of the posterior open bite.

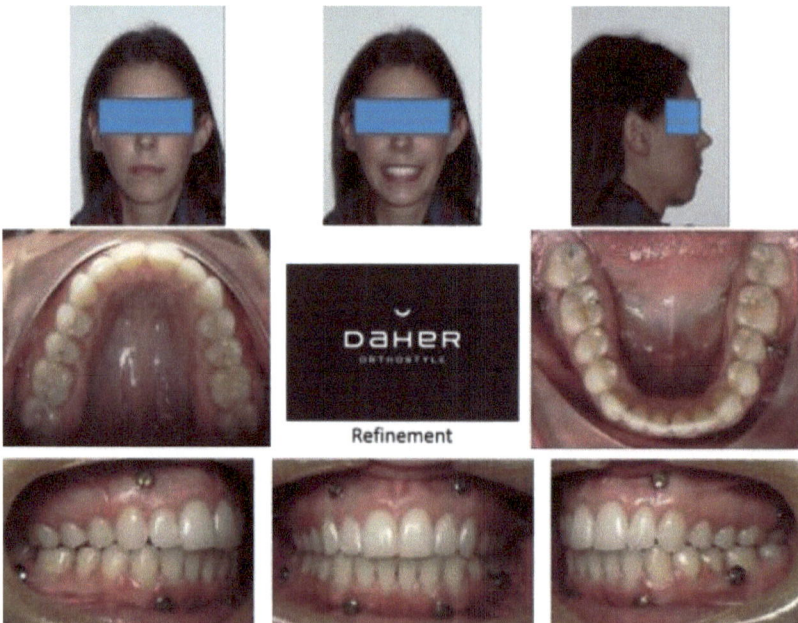

Fig. (12.21). Case 2, intraoral photos for refinement.

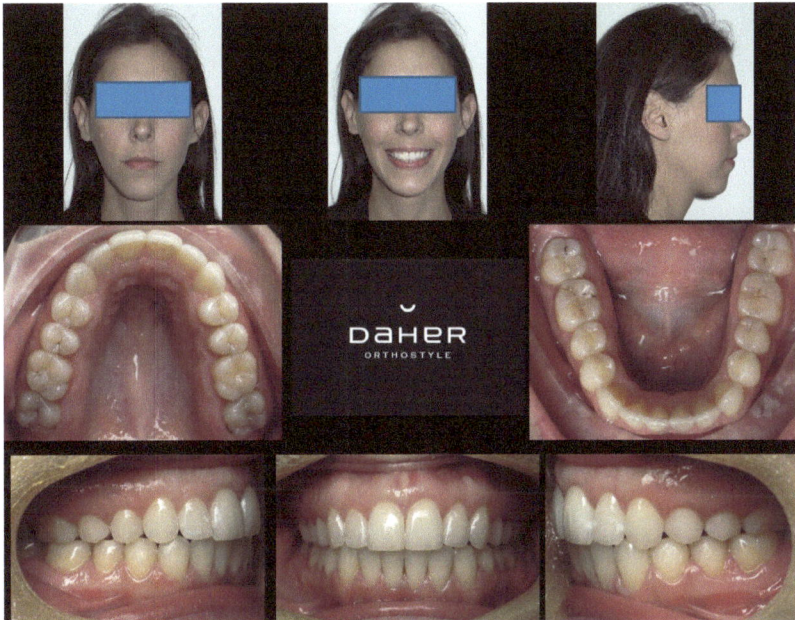

Fig. (12.22). Case 2, Final photos..

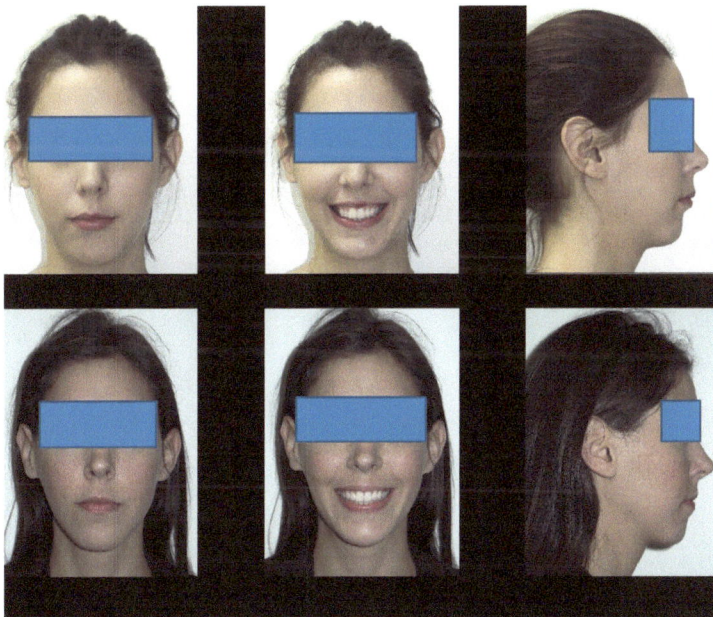

Fig. (12.23). Case 2, before and final exrtaoral photos.

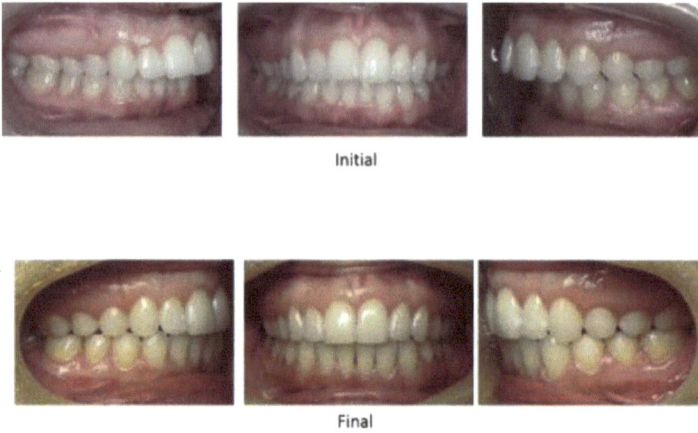

Fig. (12.24). Case 2, before and final intraoral photos.

Case 3

This is a 47-year old female presented with anterior edge to edge relationship, class III molars and canine relationship on the right side and class I molar and canine relationship on the left side (Fig. **12.25**). Lateral cephalometric radiograph confirmed the skeletal class III relationship due to maxillary deficiency (ANB =0.2°) (Fig. **12.26**).

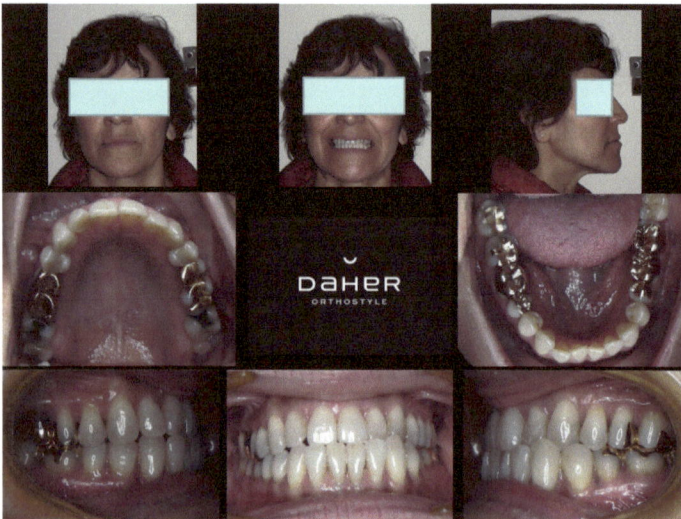

Fig. (12.25). Case 3 initial photos confirming right side class III molar and canine relationships and right first molars are in cross bite, upper midline shift to right by 2mm, anterior cross bite of 2.1,2.2,2.3 and edge to edge of 1.1. Upper and lower moderate to minimum crowding.

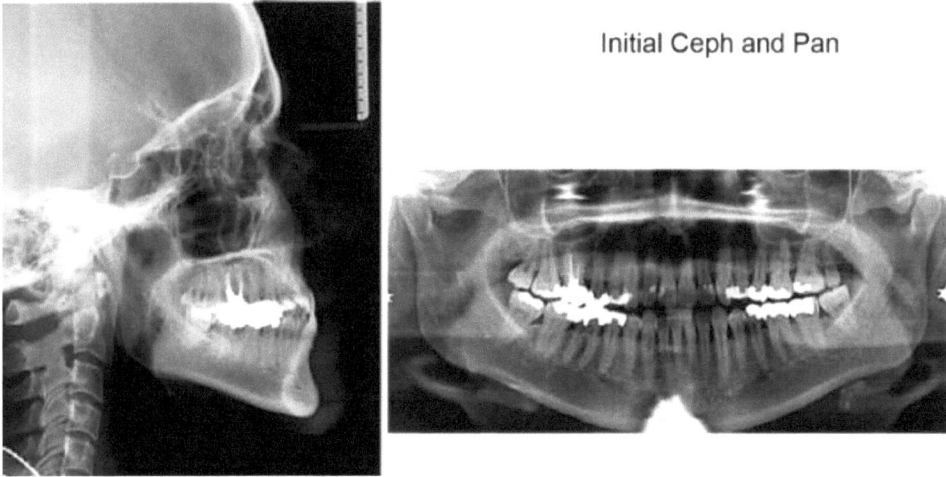

Initial Ceph and Pan

Fig. (12.26). Case 3, initial radiographs.

Treatment Objectives

1. Level and align upper and lower teeth and coordinate upper and lower arches using Invisalign;
2. Consultation for surgical maxillary advancement using Le-Forte I orthognathic surgery;
3. Finish and provide details if needed post-surgery;
4. Retention.

Treatment Progress

Patient started orthodontic treatment for leveling and alignment as well as coordinating the upper and lower arches using Invisalign treatment. Pre-surgical Invisalign consisted of upper 12 and lower 13 aligners that lead to leveling and alignment as well as coordinating upper and lower arches using lingual crown torqueing of the upper and labial crown torqueing of the lower incisors (Figs. **12.27** and **12.28**). Patient underwent LeForte I maxillary surgery with rotation to the patient's left side in order to correct the midline shift. Post-surgical records are depicted in Figs. (**12.29** and **12.30**). TADs were inserted for intermaxillary fixation as described before (Fig. **12.31**). Total treatment time including surgery lasted for 10 months. Final records are presented in Fig. (**12.32**). Before and after cephalometric radiographs (Fig. **12.33**) revealed improvement of the patient's facial profile as indicated in improvement of the ANB angle from 0.2° to +3.7°. This is confirmed by comparison of the patient's before and after profile photos (Fig. **12.34**).

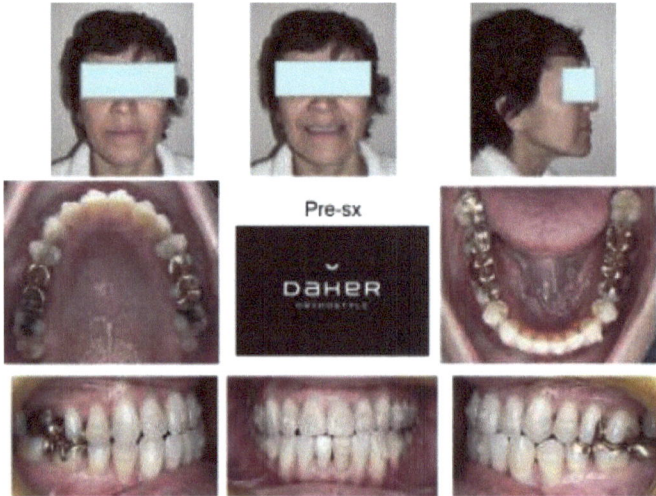

Fig. (12.27). Case 3, pre-surgical photos showing upper and lower arches are leveled, aligned and coordinated.

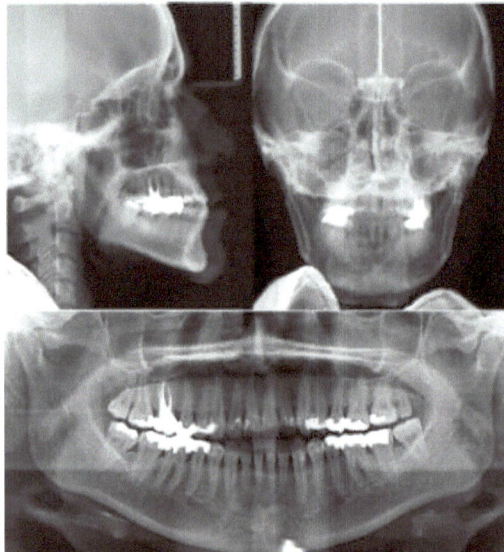

Fig. (12.28). Case 3, pre-surgical radiographs.

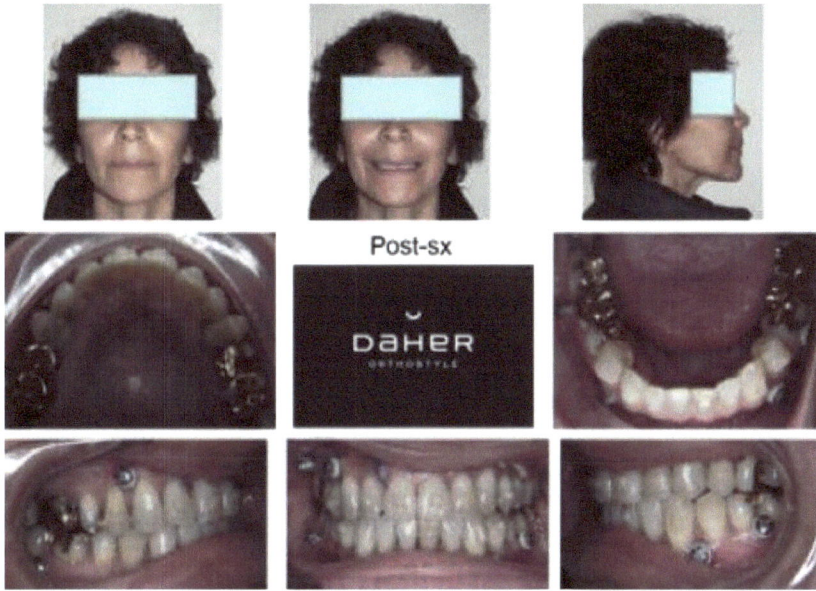

Fig. (12.29). Case 3, Post-surgical photos showing upper and lower TADs and very good occlusion.

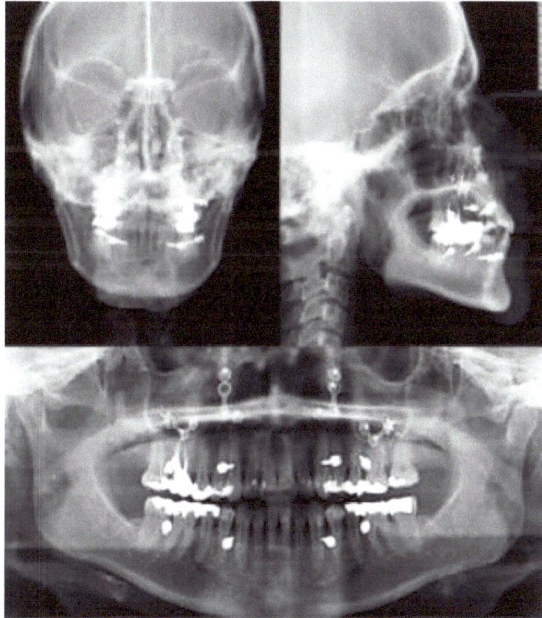

Fig. (12.30). Case 3, post-surgical radiographs showing upper and lower TADs and normal skeletal relationship as observed in the lateral cephalometric radiograph.

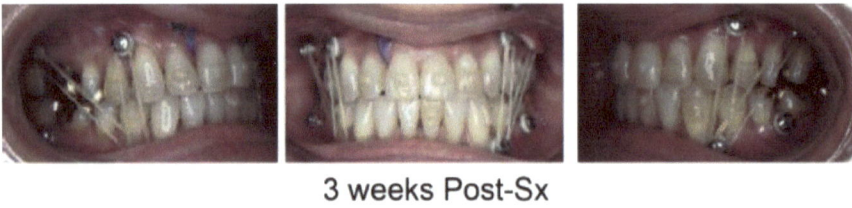

3 weeks Post-Sx

Fig. (12.31). Case 3, three weeks post-surgical radiographs showing upper and lower TADs and intermaxillary elastics.

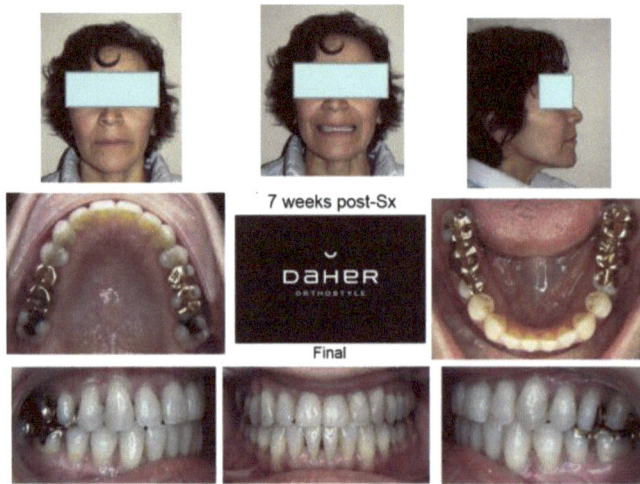

Fig. (12.32). Case 3, Final photos.

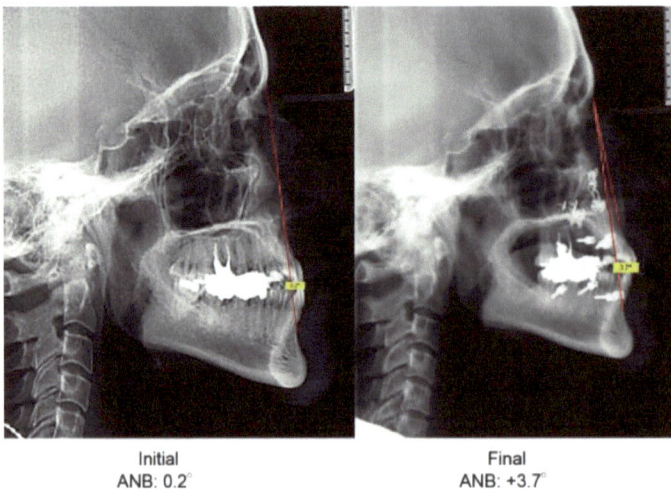

Initial
ANB: 0.2°

Final
ANB: +3.7°

Fig. (12.33). Case 3, before and after cephalometric radiographs.

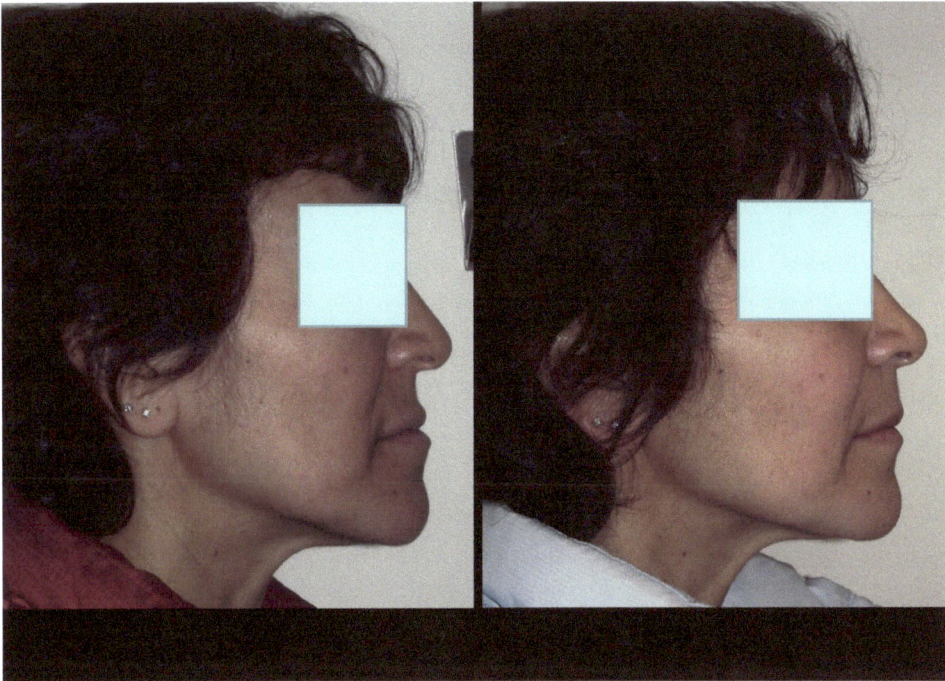

Fig. (12.34). Case 3, before and after patient's profile photographs.

SUMMARY AND CONCLUSION

Surgical orthodontic cases are feasible and the treatment time is much faster than those with regular fixed orthodontic braces. The clear aligners system is more acceptable by patients, especially adults. Healing after surgery is much faster with clear aligners as compared to those with regular fixed orthodontic braces as indicated before. Utilizing cone beam computed tomography (CBCT) is essential in these cases and would be the future in orthodontic diagnosis and treatment planning.

REFERENCES

[1]   Lu CH, Ko EW, Huang CS. The accuracy of video imaging prediction in soft tissue outcome after bimaxillary orthognathic surgery. J Oral Maxillofac Surg 2003; 61(3): 333-42.
[http://dx.doi.org/10.1053/joms.2003.50058] [PMID: 12618973]

[2]   Epker BN, Stella JP, Fish LC. Dentofacial deformities, integrated orthodontic and surgical correction. 2nd ed. St Louis, MO: Mosby Year Book 1995; p. 574.

[3]   Proffit WR, White RP. The need for surgical orthodontic treatment. St Louis, MO: Mosby Year Book

1991; p. 2.

[4]   Sarver DM, Johnston MW, Matukas VJ. Video imaging for planning and counseling in orthognathic surgery. J Oral Maxillofac Surg 1988; 46(11): 939-45.
[http://dx.doi.org/10.1016/0278-2391(88)90330-8] [PMID: 3183807]

[5]   Sarver DM, Johnston MW. Video imaging: techniques for superimposition of cephalometric radiography and profile images. Int J Adult Orthodon Orthognath Surg 1990; 5(4): 241-8.
[PMID: 2135601]

[6]   Power G, Breckon J, Sherriff M, McDonald F. Dolphin Imaging Software: an analysis of the accuracy of cephalometric digitization and orthognathic prediction. Int J Oral Maxillofac Surg 2005; 34(6): 619-26.
[http://dx.doi.org/10.1016/j.ijom.2005.04.003] [PMID: 15916879]

[7]   Lew KK. The reliability of computerized cephalometric soft tissue prediction following bimaxillary anterior subapical osteotomy. Int J Adult Orthodon Orthognath Surg 1992; 7(2): 97-101.
[PMID: 1431433]

[8]   Proffit WR, Fields HW. Contemporary Orthodontics. 3rd ed. Mosby 2000; p. 705.

[9]   Proffit W, White R Jr, Sarver D. Contemporary Treatment of Dentofacial Deformity. Mosby 2003; p. 264.

[10]   Andrews L. The six keys to normal occlusion. AmJ Orthod –DentofacOrthop 1972; 62(3): 296-309.
[http://dx.doi.org/10.1016/S0002-9416(72)90268-0] [PMID: 4505873]

[11]   Miethke RR, Brauner K. A Comparison of the periodontal health of patients during treatment with the Invisalign system and with fixed lingual appliances. J Orofac Orthop 2007; 68(3): 223-31.
[http://dx.doi.org/10.1007/s00056-007-0655-8] [PMID: 17522806]

[12]   Tawfik A, Hemeda OM, El-Bialy TH. Composite polymers transducers for ultrasonic and biological applications. Ferroelectrics Letters 2003; 30(1-2): 1-12.
[http://dx.doi.org/10.1080/713931703]

Future Directions with Clear Aligners

Future direction of clear aligners could be directed at setting up protocols that can be used in complex malocclusion cases, especially for extraction and rotation of small teeth. Materials with more stable shape memory might be introduced that are capable of producing computer animated or planned tooth movement in real situation. The implementation of CBCT in diagnosis and communication with technicians is very important. However, this would entail proper knowledge of clear aligner companies' technician to be more aware of CBCT, limitations of tooth movement and early communication with clear aligners' prescribers. Again, utilization of TADs together with clear aligners can provide an alternative treatment to difficult cases that are currently not considered candidates for clear aligners.

Recent Advances in Dentistry, 2016, *Vol. 1*, 136-138

SUBJECT INDEX

A

Aligners i, ii, 28, 30, 42, 43, 46, 48, 49, 51, 53, 68, 72, 73, 76, 78, 79, 82, 84, 86, 88, 89, 91, 98, 99, 104, 112, 115, 116, 124, 125, 129, 133, 135

Anterior open bite i, 91, 92, 94, 111

Attachments 3, 28, 34, 37, 38, 51, 52, 91, 93, 94, 98, 115

B

Basic science 8

Bio 8

Biomechanics i, iii, 6, 28, 84

Bioprogressive 51, 70, 77

Bite clearance 24, 98

Bodily 6, 33, 34, 37, 53

C

CAD 5, 8

CAM 5, 8

Camouflage 48, 78, 79, 84

Case selection 106

CBCT 13, 21, 23, 48, 51, 58, 60, 74, 76, 80, 91, 92, 101, 103, 104, 133, 135

Cephalometric 13, 45, 47, 49, 62, 63, 65, 75, 79, 81, 83, 84, 87, 88, 97, 100, 101, 103, 104, 113, 119, 122, 124, 128, 129, 131, 132, 134

Chin deviation 95, 97

Clear 13, 15, 20, 28, 30, 40, 42, 48, 51, 53, 62, 65, 73, 76, 78, 79, 84, 86, 88, 91, 94, 95, 98, 104, 133, 135

Compliance ii, 15, 26, 106

Control 3, 4, 26, 30, 58, 78, 86, 94

Cross-bite 78

Crossbite 95, 96, 103-105

D

Decalcification ii, 14, 26, 106

Decompensation 22, 79, 112, 113

Diagnosis 5, 9, 13, 22, 23, 48, 76, 78, 94, 95, 104, 112, 133, 135

Disarticulation 24

E

Early correction 24

Edge-to-edge bite 86

Effectiveness 5, 8

Elastics 38, 39, 42, 61, 62, 67, 72, 76, 77, 79, 82, 84, 89, 98, 99, 132

Expansion 40, 42, 46, 51, 96, 113, 115, 118

Extraction 5, 40, 42, 44, 45, 51, 61, 67, 88, 113, 135

Extrusion 34, 35, 86, 93, 94, 106, 118

F

Facial symmetry 15, 95

Fast 24, 76

Features i, 24

Force 10, 11, 52, 84, 91, 99

Functional shift 16, 19, 20, 103, 104

G

Growth 12, 20, 21, 23, 36, 43, 51, 53, 59, 62, 63, 67, 70, 86, 104, 107

H

Habit 86, 94

History i, 3, 14, 58, 79, 88, 96, 123

I

Interproximal 4, 40, 61, 82, 113

Intrusion 30, 34, 39, 57, 75, 86, 91

Tarek El-Bialy, Donna Galante & Sam Daher

X   X-ray 13, 19, 20, 65

www.ingramcontent.com/pod-product-compliance
Lightning Source LLC
Chambersburg PA
CBHW041714210326

41598CB00007B/646